Beyond Cholesterol

Beyond Cholesterol

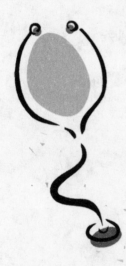

7 Life-Saving

Heart Disease Tests

That Your Doctor

May Not Give You

JULIUS TORELLI, M.D.
with George Ryan
A Lynn Sonberg Book

 St. Martin's Griffin ≋ New York

www.stmartins.com

Library of Congress Cataloging-in-Publication Data

Torelli, Julius.
    Beyond cholesterol: 7 life-saving heart disease tests that your doctor
 may not give you / Julius Torelli with George Ryan.
        p. cm.
    ISBN 0-312-34863-0
    EAN 978-0-312-34863-2
    1. Coronary heart disease—Prevention—Popular works. 2. Cho-
lesterol—Health aspects. I. Ryan, George. II. Title.

RC685.C6T547 2005
616.1'2305—dc22   2005045288

First Edition: October 2005

10   9   8   7   6   5   4   3   2   1

Important Note

This book is for informational purposes only. It is not intended to take the place of medical or nutritional advice from a trained health-care professional. Readers are advised to consult a physician or other qualified health professional regarding all concerns related to heart health and before making any changes to their diet.

Contents

Part II. The Essential New Tests

Introduction

In my residency and training as a young physician, I learned how to use high technology to treat ailing people. In early practice, I worked with highly trained doctors and focused on symptoms and illnesses. Under pressure, we could work as efficiently and smoothly as a MASH unit. We put sick or injured people on their feet again and sent them on their way. Only later did it occur to me that the kind of medicine we concentrated on—and did very well—was only part of the whole picture. We excelled at treating what are called acute problems, that is, short-term disorders requiring a quick fix. We received much less training in dealing with chronic health problems and consequently had much less success in treating them.

A good doctor is unlikely to be a comic-book hero who zaps textbook diseases in anonymous patients with brand-name drugs. In real life, much of a good doctor's practice involves helping people with long-term and sometimes multiple health problems. The doctor can show patients how to alleviate their suffering and prevent complications and new illnesses from developing. Having heart disease, needless to say, is a long-term health problem. As doctors get to know their patients, they almost invariably learn how much patients' lifestyles and personalities are involved with their health.

In 1999, I founded a heart clinic, called the Integrative Cardiology Center, in High Point, North Carolina, to make use of high technology and research in conjunction with lifestyle change and emotional issues. At the clinic, we take a holistic approach to patients—your whole body matters, not just the ailing part of your cardiovascular system. Besides conventional medical approaches, we provide Asian medicine, yoga, and massage therapy. And, very important, we listen to our patients.

The Integrative Cardiology Center has been a great success. As it grew, I became busier and less active and found my weight harder to control. As I became busier and busier, I had more and more stress. I had less time for my family. I had no time for exercise. I knew I shouldn't be behaving like this and intended to slow down when I had some time. I never found any. One day, I had chest pain. I was having a heart attack. I was 42.

This scenario happens more often with doctors than you might imagine. We tend to have a strong drive, there are always more sick people than doctors can manage, and we can work ourselves to death. I am aware of the irony of a cardiologist working himself to the point of a heart attack in his own heart clinic. I am telling you, as I tell some of my patients: It happened to me; don't let it happen to you.

As a cardiologist, I see the heart and blood circulation as my area of special expertise. But unlike a traditional specialist, I am acutely aware at all times how other body systems and organs have to be taken into account while dealing with the cardiovascular system. The regulation of blood sugar level by the hormone insulin is a good example of how various organs and systems work in balance. Keeping the body's systems in working balance is one way to define the maintenance of good health.

Balance is key. One way to measure balance is through lab tests on a blood sample. When the blood level of some special substance (for example, fibrinogen or homocysteine) is too high or too low—out of balance—something is not working as it's supposed to. On the other hand, when the blood level of that substance is within normal range, that bodily system is probably in balance.

The fact that one particular substance is in balance doesn't mean that everything all over the body is in good working shape, because some substances are better indicators of a system's health than others. Additionally, some substances are more readily obtainable and easier to test. The ability to measure overall health changes with advances in testing, but much depends on whether the tests are put into use—and how effectively.

When a new test substance (such as C-reactive protein) proves reliable, practical, and cost-effective for daily clinical use, some doctors respond more quickly than others. Or well-informed patients may demand a new test before their doctors have familiarized themselves with it. It's important to keep in mind that the new test substance is not new in the sense of being newly discovered, and the test it is being used in is not new either. What is new is the availability of the test to ordinary people at a reasonable cost. This book will explain seven such new cardiac tests.

There is a need for new cardiac tests, because while we once believed that cholesterol tests told us almost everything we needed to know, we now know better. Cholesterol tests provide valuable information, but they don't tell the whole story. In fact, they leave out some really important aspects. Acting as if this one piece of information presents the whole story can put your health at risk.

Six of the seven new tests in this book tell you as much of the whole story of your heart as you can obtain by walking into your doctor's office and giving a blood sample. They fill the gaps in the story left by conventional lab tests.

In addition to the new tests, we look at emerging information on conventional blood tests. Although some knowledge has been around for a while, it still has to find its way into everyday medical practice. Some long familiar assumptions are seen differently when viewed from a new perspective. For example, low-density lipoprotein (LDL) cholesterol level has lost much of its luster as a *predictor* of heart attacks, but is seen increasingly as the most important blood lipid level in therapy.

We look at the issue of low-carb versus low-fat diets and some of the confusions over dieting, as well as why we have weight problems in the United States today. You will see that you don't need to lose nearly as much weight to be healthy as you do to be beautiful. A key component for health is to be active for at least a half hour every day. You will see that this can be fun, not a burden.

This book contains the information you need to determine how healthy your heart is. It will also show you how to look in a new way at some things you thought you knew all about. The bottom line is that only you can protect your heart. Here is the way to do it.

Part I

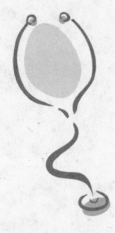

The Heart of the Matter

Our Understanding
of Heart Disease
Continues to Evolve

1. A New Look at Heart Disease

Cardiovascular disease" is a catchall term for diseases of the heart and blood vessels, or the vascular system. Coronary artery disease (also called "coronary heart disease") is the usual cause of heart attacks and the most frequent kind of cardiovascular disease. Other kinds include stroke, high blood pressure, and arrhythmia (irregular heartbeat).

Your heart pumps blood to every part of your body through a network of blood vessels. The heart pumps the blood through thicker-walled arteries, and the blood returns to the heart through thinner-walled veins. The blood carries glucose and oxygen, the fuel for your cells.

Your coronary arteries lie on the surface of your heart and supply it with blood that has been freshly oxygenated by the lungs. Your heart, which is almost entirely composed of muscle, depends on a generous supply of this arterial blood for its ceaseless activity.

If something—such as a blockage to one or more coronary arteries—interferes with this blood supply to any part of the heart, that hard-working section of muscle is deprived of oxygen and nutrients, and the cells quickly die. This process is a heart attack.

Causes of Deaths from
Cardiovascular Disease in 2001

Coronary artery disease	54%
Stroke	18%
Heart failure	6%
High blood pressure	5%
Others	17%

SOURCE: Centers for Disease Control and Prevention.

Heart's Blood

The heart is a nonstop muscular pump that drives blood through your body with the force of its contractions. It has four chambers. The upper two, called "atria," are filling chambers. The lower two, called "ventricles," are pumping chambers. Each upper and lower chamber is connected by a one-way-flow valve, but there are no connections between the right and left chambers. Thus the heart is divided in two, the right side pumping oxygen-poor blood from the body to the lungs, and the left side pumping oxygen-rich blood to the body. To get from the right side of the heart to its left side, the blood has to pass through a second smaller circulation system between the heart and the lungs.

The oxygen-poor blood, returning from the body through the veins, enters the heart through the upper right chamber, or atrium. As the heart relaxes, the right atrium blood is sucked down through the tricuspid valve into the right ventricle. With succeeding

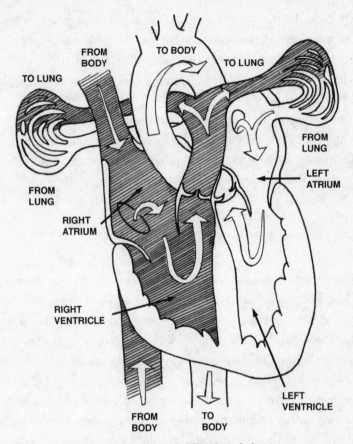

Direction of blood flow through the
heart's chambers. (Illustration by Caspar Henselmann.)

contractions, this blood is forced from the heart to the lungs and
into tiny vessels in the lung linings, where it is oxygenated by coming into contact with the air you breathe.

The oxygenated blood is pumped back to the left side of the
heart. It enters the left atrium, passes through the mitral valve
down into the left ventricle, and leaves the heart through the mas-
sive artery called the aorta. The aorta carries blood to arteries all
over the body. The right and left coronary arteries branch off the

aorta close to the heart's surface, on which they progressively branch farther. As they do elsewhere in the body, these arteries branch until they form a network of capillaries embedded in the tissues, where the exchange of oxygen and carbon dioxide with the cells takes place.

A buildup of fatty material in the wall of a coronary artery is called atherosclerosis. This buildup often requires decades before it narrows the interior (lumen) of the artery. The entire process of this buildup is termed "coronary artery disease."

Inside a Coronary Artery

Coronary artery disease begins with the cells that line the inside wall of a coronary artery. This cell layer is called the "endothelium." Fatty material and other debris, called "plaque," build up in the middle wall of the artery. As the plaque grows, it stretches the endothelium, subsequently narrowing the space for blood to flow through. Until a few years ago, the plaque was thought to build up inside the artery until it completely obstructed blood flow. A comparison was frequently made to deposits lining a water pipe building up to the extent that they block flow. Because cholesterol makes up a good part of the fatty material in plaque, it seemed reasonable to assume that people with a high total blood cholesterol level are at high risk of developing plaque on the insides of their coronary arteries, and they are. But, as was discovered in time, many people with normal total cholesterol levels also develop coronary artery disease. In addition, many people with high cholesterol levels never develop heart trouble. Doctors came to realize that cholesterol is not the whole story. It seems that other important factors are involved.

Doctors offered a new explanation, based on new research and clinicians' observations of their heart patients. Plaque had been assumed to be inactive debris, these doctors pointed out. Although plaque contains fragments of fatty materials and calcium as well as dead cells, much of it is composed of various kinds of white blood cells and smooth muscle cells. In other words, the plaque inside coronary arteries is not lifeless debris encrusted on the inside of a pipe, but a form of tissue capable of change in response to its surroundings.

So what happens? What causes plaque to form? And why does it form on one part of an inside wall and not on another? Doctors don't yet have all the answers, but they do have some of them. We will look now at how researchers think the whole process of atherosclerosis begins.

Attack on the Artery Wall

Dr. Russell Ross of the University of Washington School of Medicine in Seattle pioneered the new approach to atherosclerosis. Following is a highly simplified account of the process.

As in a flowing stream, forks, branches, and curves in an artery increase the turbulence and the sheer stress of flowing blood. It is at such sites that plaque builds, particularly when something alters the blood flow. Although we focus on coronary arteries because they are the arteries involved in heart attacks, plaque can occur in any artery. In the coronary arteries of people who are vulnerable for whatever reason, three processes get under way. These three processes are the predecessors of plaque buildup, which ultimately develops into atherosclerosis.

1. The cells lining the artery wall increasingly allow fatty particles and other substances in the bloodstream to

pass through their walls into their interiors.

2. Adhesion molecules cling to cells lining the artery wall. These adhesion molecules cause white blood cells to adhere and gather. The white blood cell types are usually monocytes and T cells. Other substances are involved, including modified low-density lipoprotein (LDL).

3. LDL and other substances enable the white blood cells to migrate into the artery wall.

These three processes that make up the beginnings of atherosclerosis are a long way from the concept of sediment encrusting the inside of a pipe. The living cells involved in these three processes secrete substances that affect other cells in their vicinity. The secreting cells in turn are controlled by other substances, such as enzymes, the origins of which in some cases can be traced back to genes or to a person's physical condition or lifestyle.

So, even before plaque begins to form, we see that certain artery wall cells change, permitting fatty substances to enter them, allowing adhesion molecules and white blood cells to attach to them, and letting modified white blood cells, helped by LDL, migrate into the cell wall lining. Whatever initiates these three processes can be credited with beginning coronary artery disease. Needless to say, doctors are looking closely at possible candidates. For Dr. Ross, the following are high-ranking contenders:

- High LDL blood level
- Presence of modified LDL particles in bloodstream
- Free radicals caused by cigarette smoking, high blood pressure, and diabetes

- High homocysteine blood level
- Products of infectious microorganisms such as herpes-viruses, *Chlamydia pneumoniae,* and *Nanobacterium sanguiniem*
- Combinations of these or other factors

Foam Cells and Fatty Streaks

We mentioned that white blood cells usually arrive at the artery wall site in the form of monocytes and T cells. Monocytes can morph into large scavenger cells called "macrophages," which engulf invaders in video-game style. LDL particles are a favorite prey. Macrophage and LDL together are known as a "foam cell."

Foam cells, monocytes laden with fatty substances, and T cells together form a fatty streak in the artery wall. These cells are later joined by smooth muscle cells from the cell layer beneath. Fatty streaks are found in the arteries of people of all ages, including very young children. They have been seen at autopsy in the coronary arteries of fetuses whose mothers had very high cholesterol levels.

On the inside artery wall, sticky platelets adhere. Platelets are a kind of blood cell that helps in the formation of clots.

The presence of LDL is thought to be responsible for the change of monocytes into macrophages. The whole process of foam cell and fatty streak formation is an inflammatory process. In inflammation, white blood cells arrive to defend against the attackers, which the immune system assumes are invaders from outside the body. In this case, things go wrong and pathological conditions develop. Keep in mind that this can be a very long, drawn-out process in a person's arteries, extending over many years or even decades.

Plaque Formation

If the inflammatory process does not neutralize or get rid of the agents causing injury to the cells lining the artery wall, the inflammation can go on indefinitely. We know that the inflammatory process causes smooth muscle cells from the cell layer beneath the wall-lining cells to mix and multiply among the monocytes, foam cells, and T cells of the lesion. As the inflammation continues, the lesion gets bigger. The artery wall thickens. The artery compensates for this by dilating, thus keeping its lumen from narrowing. So long as this compensation takes place, the blood flow is unimpeded.

Once expansion of the artery can no longer compensate for the increasing size of the lesion, the lesion begins to bulge into the artery lumen. In time, with continuing inflammation, the bulge progressively narrows the arterial lumen and slows down blood flow.

As a fatty streak grows into a bulging lesion, it usually becomes covered with a fibrous cap that separates the contents of the lesion from the blood in the arterial lumen. You can think of this fibrous cap as being equivalent to a scab forming over an open cut. The cap covers a mixture of various kinds of white blood cells, fatty substances, calcium fragments, and dead cells— what we call plaque. Fat particles and dead cells often form a necrotic core.

Blocking of the Coronary Artery

Stable plaque with a uniformly dense fibrous cap does not present an immediate cardiac threat. If the plaque is not growing and permits sufficient quantities of blood to flow through the artery, the status quo can be maintained for many years. However, in an angiogram it's very difficult to tell stable plaque with a dense cap from unstable plaque with a thin cap. Enzymes secreted by macrophages are thought to thin the fibrous cap, and thinning of the fibrous cap can result in rupture. Concentrations of macrophages seem to be denser at rupture sites. High blood levels of fibrinogen and C-reactive protein may indicate an accumulation of macrophages.

When the fibrous cap ruptures, the plaque interior comes in contact with the arterial blood and a clot forms. This blood clot is what usually blocks the coronary artery, resulting in a lack of supply of oxygenated blood to a section of heart muscle cells and a consequent heart attack. If the resulting clot does not completely block the artery, but rather causes an 80 to 90 percent narrowing, unstable angina may result. The area of rupture then slowly heals and the blockage may shrink to perhaps 50 percent of its former size. This may then occur over and over again. The whole process is very dynamic.

Until recently, it was assumed that a cholesterol-based plaque grew and grew until it reached such a size in the lumen of the artery that it blocked the flow of blood. Under these circumstances, demonizing cholesterol is understandable. Now we know better. Yes, cholesterol is extremely important in plaque buildup, especially in the form of LDL. But cholesterol levels are not the best indicators of the likelihood of fibrous cap rupture and a subsequent blood clot that blocks the coronary artery, causing a heart attack. C-reactive protein and fibrinogen blood levels may be the best indicators of that possibility.

Symptoms of Heart Attack

Many people imagine that those who are having a heart attack clutch their chest, grimace, roll their eyes, and fall down. When this happens, it is not caused directly by the heart attack but often by a ventricular fibrillation. This is an arrhythmia of the heart (a form of heart failure) that can occur at the same time as, or shortly after, a heart attack. During ventricular fibrillation, the heart is actually beating so fast (at more than 600 beats per minute) that there is no significant contraction of the pumping chamber. The chamber is quivering rather than contracting.

The symptoms of a heart attack are quite different:

- Pressure, tightness, heaviness, or squeezing in the chest
- Arm discomfort (usually in the left arm)
- Burning sensation in the stomach or chest

These are the typical or so-called classical symptoms. Half the people having heart attacks have at least some of them. Another quarter of the people have what are called "atypical symptoms"— they feel tired or nauseated, or they feel pain in a body part not closely linked to the heart. And the final quarter have "silent" heart attacks—they have no prior symptoms and often do not know what is happening to them.

A Heart Attack

Heart attacks occur most frequently in the early morning between the hours of 5:00 A.M. and 9:00 A.M. In climates with a cold winter, that's the season when most heart attacks take place.

In medical language, a heart attack is an acute myocardial infarction. The myocardium is the heart muscle. An infarct is an area of dead tissue (necrosis) caused by lack of blood supply. Nearly all heart attacks are caused by coronary disease. The heart muscle cells dependent on the blocked coronary artery begin to die about thirty minutes after complete blockage occurs. If the blood supply is not restored to that part of the heart within three to six hours, about 90 percent of the muscle cells will die. That is the window of opportunity for saving the cells. Once they die, they are replaced by scar tissue in the heart of a survivor. The dead cells are never replaced by new cells in an effective way. How much someone's heart is permanently damaged by a heart attack depends on the amount of cells affected.

The pain of a heart attack varies with individuals. Typically you feel chest heaviness, burning, tightness, or pressure. You may also feel dizzy, weak, or short of breath, find yourself sweating, and perhaps have nausea and vomiting. If your discomfort is unfamiliar to you, you may indeed be having a heart attack. You need urgent help.

Because of the small window of opportunity to restore the blood supply to the affected heart muscle cells, you need to take action. It is best to have a friend take you to the hospital emergency room or call an ambulance.

2. Coronary Artery Disease Risk Factors

Atherosclerosis—the buildup of plaque in the walls of coronary arteries—is a very slow process, often extending over decades. In autopsies on accident fatalities, pathologists regularly find atherosclerosis well under way in the coronary arteries of men and women in their twenties. They also find it in obese teenagers. Atherosclerosis is slow, it's insidious, and it starts early. A man who has a heart attack at 50 may have had, without knowing it, coronary artery disease since he was 20.

Don't wait until your forties or fifties before you become concerned about your cardiac health. If you do, you are giving atherosclerosis a possible head start of twenty or thirty years. You need to start early and take preventive measures all your life.

Things that directly cause or indirectly contribute to the development of atherosclerosis are known as "coronary artery disease risk factors." Neil Schneiderman and colleagues at the University of Miami arranged these risk factors into three groups. The first group is composed of risk factors that have been proven to be direct causes.

- Cigarette smoking
- High blood cholesterol levels
- High blood pressure
- Advancing age

The second group is made up of risk factors that without doubt are associated with coronary artery disease but whose mode of operation is less certain.

- High blood triglyceride levels
- Coagulation factors
- Certain lipoproteins
- Homocysteine

The third group consists of risk factors that are probably not direct causes of atherosclerosis but make people vulnerable to it. These risk factors can interact with those above to heighten the risk.

- Obesity
- Sedentary lifestyle
- Family history of coronary artery disease
- Male gender
- Insulin resistance
- Psychosocial factors

We should never expect a single cause-and-effect relationship between these risk factors and coronary artery disease. Risk factors usually don't act alone and they need to be triggered. When you have two or more risk factors, they can interact synergistically. Besides, individuals differ so much and in so many ways, something harmful to one person may be harmless to another. For example, some people smoke all their lives and have no ill effects. Possibly they have genes to protect them from the toxins in tobacco smoke. Or they may not have the gene for coronary artery disease. While your genes may protect you from some risky behavior, chances are that they will not. You may not be one of the lucky few.

Homocysteine is listed above as a risk factor. Some doctors would disagree and consider it only a marker or indicator of coronary artery disease. The same is true for C-reactive protein. Some consider it a marker and others a risk factor. With a risk factor, the implication is that the substance itself is harmful. With a marker or indicator, the substance itself is probably more or less harmless, but it acts as a signal that something is happening. For us, this issue is irrelevant. We know that when levels are too high, we need to lower them. From the patient's point of view, the resolution of scientific questions is of secondary importance. The question that needs to be foremost in your mind is: Can this help without harming me?

• GREG'S STORY •

Until he turned 30, Greg never put on a pound of extra weight, no matter what or how much he ate or drank. But at 30, he now remembers, his metabolism seemed to slow down. Over the years since then, his body chemistry seemed to get progressively slower. Today, at 47, Greg jokes that he has only to *think* of beer and pizza to put on weight.

Greg's wife sees things differently. She says he didn't take care of his body, wouldn't listen to her, and now has middle-age spread. Men much older than him who looked after themselves are in much better shape. According to her, Greg has no one to blame but himself.

Greg doesn't argue. But he says that if things were as simple as his wife makes them sound, his efforts to help himself would have shown more results. He feels trapped by a general feeling of unwellness. In addition, he has a job that he hates and that does not pay him enough money. He feels as though he needs to work sixty hours or more per week and is too tired and depressed to exercise. This lowers his metabolism further, which causes additional weight gain.

He claims he has found a new way to control his high blood pressure and high cholesterol—don't get tested anymore.

Greg is less original than he thinks. Denial is the way many people, particularly men, cope with health challenges. Saying that ill health is an inevitable result of getting older is another common excuse for doing nothing. Unfortunately, Greg has the metabolic syndrome, as people with a medical history like his often do.

• • •

Finding Your Way in the Metabolic Syndrome Maze

The metabolic syndrome was named "syndrome X" by its discoverer, Dr. Gerald Reaven of Stanford University. It's also widely known as "insulin resistance syndrome." The syndrome's definition tends to vary with the professional viewpoint of the person discussing it.

The syndrome, as Dr. Reaven originally conceived it, consisted of the following:

- Insulin resistance
- High insulin blood level
- High total cholesterol blood level
- High blood pressure
- Glucose intolerance
- Small LDL particle size
- High triglyceride blood level
- High level of triglyceride-rich remnant lipoproteins after meals
- Low HDL blood level
- Increased risk of diabetes
- Increased risk of coronary artery disease

Not even Greg had *all* these problems. There are differing viewpoints on how many of these problems you need to have, and which ones, in order to qualify for the syndrome. The metabolic syndrome is really a collection of health problems that can interact with one another to form a powerful threat to the heart. Any two or three of the problems acting together are far more potent than one alone. When you seem to get a handle on one problem, others begin to act up.

The metabolic syndrome has been associated with dysfunction of the cells lining the interior artery wall. The syndrome has also been connected to increased numbers of adhesion molecules circulating in the bloodstream. We talked about these adhesion molecules in Chapter 1.

Of the five new tests that I recommend in this book, the inflammatory markers C-reactive protein and fibrinogen are also indicators of metabolic syndrome.

According to Dr. Reaven, metabolic syndrome is fundamentally due to high insulin blood levels as a result of insulin resistance. Of the five tests, the fasting insulin test is a good indicator of metabolic syndrome. A lab test result of more than 15 is indicative of the syndrome.

Metabolic Syndrome Indicators

C-reactive protein level	High
Fibrinogen level	High
Insulin level	More than 15
Triglyceride level	More than 200
Triglyceride/HDL ratio	More than 3

An important aspect of understanding the metabolic syndrome is that it introduces us to the concept that risk factors don't come alone and they are dangerous to ignore. To handle them, you usually need professional help. Ask your doctor if you need medication for high blood pressure or high cholesterol.

Besides seeking the advice of your doctor, I can only tell you what I told Greg: Lead a more active life and trim your waistline. A sedentary lifestyle leads to obesity and then to the metabolic syndrome. Increased activity and weight loss greatly improve insulin resistance and subsequently lessen the symptoms of the metabolic syndrome.

3. Women's Heart Risks

In February 2004, the American Heart Association (AHA) issued new guidelines to help women prevent heart attacks and strokes. (To contact the AHA, phone 1-888-MYHEART.) According to AHA records, about 40,000 American women died of breast cancer in 2003, while more than ten times that number of women died of heart attacks and strokes. Even so, American women remain focused on the threat of breast cancer and continue to be relatively oblivious about cardiovascular disease. Over the past two decades, more American women than men have died of heart disease. While there has been a 12 percent decrease in men's deaths from heart disease over that period, the rate for women has remained steady. Despite these facts, many women persist in their belief that heart disease is a male problem.

An AHA survey, issued with the guidelines, of more than a thousand women found the following:

- More than 50 percent knew that cardiovascular disease is the number one killer of women.
- Only 13 percent believed that they personally were at risk.
- Less than 30 percent knew their cholesterol level or blood pressure.

In an earlier study by L. Pilote and M. A. Hlatky at McGill University in Montreal, three out of four women considered their risk of coronary artery disease by the age of 70 to be only 1 in 100. Of those women, a third thought their risk to be only 1 in 1,000.

Here are some of the American Heart Association guidelines for women to prevent heart attacks and strokes:

- Women need to begin taking preventive-care measures by the age of 20.
- Even when their LDL level is normal, women at *high* cardiac risk should consider taking a cholesterol-lowering drug.
- Women should not seek cardiac protection from hormone replacement therapy.
- With a blood pressure of 140/90 or above, women should take a blood pressure–lowering drug or consider other methods of lowering their blood pressure.
- Women at low cardiac risk should not take daily aspirin as a preventive measure, because the benefit is outweighed by the risk of stroke, bleeding, and stomach problems.

At 60 years of age, 1 in 17 women has had a coronary event, compared to 1 in 5 men. Over the age of 60, on the other hand, the death rate from coronary artery disease is 1 in 4 for both women and men. Because women generally get heart attacks a decade later in age than men, and because they have a higher risk for heart attack after menopause, the female hormone estrogen has been assumed to have a protective role. For many years, it was also assumed that hormone replacement therapy provided cardiac protection. We now know that this is untrue. Most gynecologists today do not recommend hormone replacement therapy, except in cases of severe menopause symptoms. When hormone replacement therapy is justified by the severity of the symptoms a woman is suffering, they are recommended to restrict the therapy to six months or less.

Rather than having a *protective* role, estrogen has a *delaying* role. Women and men have the same risks for heart disease—except that women generally suffer the consequences ten years later than men. While this gives women ten added years free of cardiac trouble, when trouble finally comes they are ten years older and their powers of recovery are weaker. In addition, women's blood vessels are smaller, so that it takes less plaque to potentially cause problems.

Dr. Nanette Kass Wenger, a professor of medicine at Emory University School of Medicine in Atlanta, summarized the facts in this way:

- After menopause, a woman has a 31 percent lifetime chance of dying from coronary artery disease, against a 3 percent chance from breast cancer or hip fracture.
- Of women 45 to 54 years of age, one in eight has symptoms of coronary artery disease.
- Of women over 65, one in three has symptoms of coronary artery disease.
- Of people hospitalized for a heart attack, 16 percent of women and 11 percent of men die.
- A year after a heart attack, fewer women than men survive.

- Because she is likely to have so many risk factors for heart disease, almost any American woman can greatly benefit from taking cardiac protective measures.

• JENNIFER'S STORY •

Jennifer had always been one of the best women golfers in the state of Ohio. Even now, although she had turned 59, the only women who could beat her were college players being trained by pros. Her husband traveled a lot on business. Having no children or job, she put in time on the fairways and greens almost every day. That was her life. She had no complaints.

While she played, Jennifer began to notice a heaviness deep inside her chest. When she stopped being active, the discomfort slowly disappeared. She avoided spicy food and took an antacid, which didn't seem to make much difference. She couldn't help noticing that the more active she was, the worse the discomfort became. Without saying anything to her husband, she made an appointment to see her doctor.

He told her that she might have angina pectoris and sent her to a cardiologist. The cardiologist took her history and performed a physical examination, electrocardiogram, and exercise echocardiogram. These confirmed that a plaque had built up on an artery's interior wall, causing obstruction to blood flow. She had coronary artery disease. Her angina was caused by muscle cells being starved of oxygen as a result of the obstruction in the artery.

"I don't smoke," she said. "I never have more than two drinks. I'm fit. It's not fair."

"Has anyone in your family had heart trouble?" the cardiologist asked.

"My father died of a heart attack when he was younger than I am now," she answered. "My older brother has had two. But they never took care of themselves. I have."

Nonetheless the tests suggested blockage.

• • •

Angina: A Warning Signal

Angina is a warning signal. (All too often, particularly for men, the first symptom of coronary artery disease is a heart attack, which may be fatal.) Angina is frequently described not as pain, but as a tightness or heaviness. In fact, most people with angina deny having pain. They usually say they feel heaviness, "like an elephant sitting on my chest." If you feel chest discomfort only when you are active, as Jennifer did, that usually means a coronary artery is at least 60 to 70 percent narrowed. If the discomfort changes or lasts longer, the coronary artery has likely become unstable. But angina differs widely among individuals. Additionally, emotional stress and physical stresses like cold weather can bring on angina. But you can't depend on angina as a warning signal. No pain at all is felt in "silent" coronary artery disease.

On feeling the discomfort of angina, people can incorrectly assume that they are actually having a heart attack. Notoriously, indigestion can cause a discomfort similar to angina. So too can anxiety or a panic attack. A gallbladder problem can also be responsible.

A spasm can restrict blood flow through a coronary artery and result in angina. Spasms seem to occur more often in coronary arteries already narrowed by plaque buildup. The combination of spasm and plaque can greatly reduce the blood flow, causing intense discomfort.

Artery walls need to expand and contract with blood flow. When the walls lose this flexibility, angina can result. It is believed that microvascular angina is caused by the inability of tiny blood vessels to conduct blood normally.

People can live into old age with angina. When they exert themselves to a certain degree, they develop chest pain. They know their limits, and although they are not getting better, they are not getting worse. Their angina is stable. But once people notice that they develop chest pain with less physical effort than before or that the discomfort lasts longer, they have *unstable* angina. This can mean that their coronary arteries are becoming increasingly narrowed or that the plaque has ruptured but the resulting blood clots have not blocked off the artery completely. Unstable angina is a danger signal that must not be ignored. They need to see a doctor without delay. Unstable angina is frequently a precursor of a heart attack.

Women's Chest Pain

Chest pain is a frequent complaint of women. Their doctors often refer them to cardiologists to be sure the pain is not of cardiac origin. An arteriogram is the most reliable way to check whether the cardiovascular system is involved, but this is an invasive and expensive procedure. A radioopaque dye is injected into the circulating blood and its progress is followed on a monitor. This does not show the plaque, but rather the obstruction in the lumen of the artery. Its risks include the rare occurrence of kidney damage or a stroke. How frequently is a woman's chest pain found to be a symptom of heart disease? Is her chest pain the same symptom as a man's? To answer such questions, researchers reviewed the results for patients of one British cardiologist for the years 1987 to 1991. These patients were all women who had been referred for chest pain and who had received an arteriogram.

The researchers, from the Royal Brompton National Heart and Lung Hospital in London and the London Chest Hospital, led by A. K. Sullivan, followed up on the women's health for several years. They found the following:

- Women frequently feel chest pain, but it is often not a symptom of heart trouble.
- Chest pain in a woman is not the same symptom as in a man.
- Of the women, 41 percent had normal coronary arteries. Of men with chest pain who had an arteriogram, only 8 percent turned out to have normal coronary arteries.
- Risk factors and simple EKG stress tests may not be as diagnostically reliable for women as men.
- Many of the women whose coronary arteries proved to be normal did not accept the diagnosis and continued to request medication for angina.

Because women have frequently been excluded or included only in small numbers in cardiac research projects, doctors often find it hard to know if all the tests and treatments that apply to men also apply to women. For example, if the testing of a new heart disease drug has been done mostly on men, should doctors assume the drug will have the same effects on women? No, they shouldn't, according to Dr. Pamela Douglas and Dr. Geoffrey Ginsburg of Harvard Medical School and Beth Israel Hospital in Boston. They point out that women with stable angina are more likely than men to have chest pain under stress or while resting or sleeping. Chest pain occurring at rest in men is unlikely to be caused by coronary artery disease, but this is not the case in women.

However, women are even more likely than men to suffer from "silent" coronary artery disease, that is, with no symptoms. In the famous Framingham Heart Study, nearly two-thirds of the women who died suddenly of coronary artery disease had no symptoms, in contrast to about half of the men.

Hospital Treatment of Women Heart Patients

Responding to widespread complaints that women heart attack victims received poorer hospital treatment than men, researchers investigated the university and city hospitals of Nottingham, in the English Midlands. K. W. Clarke and the University of Nottingham researchers decided that the women's chances of survival were not as good as the men's because their treatment was not as good, both in the hospital and after discharge. What happens in England, of course, may not happen in the United States, but here are their main findings:

- It took longer for women heart attack victims to arrive at the hospital than for men.
- Women were less likely to be admitted directly to the coronary care unit and therefore less likely to get timely clot-dissolving treatment.
- Women's heart attacks were generally more serious than men's.
- On admission to the hospital with a heart attack, women had a slightly higher death rate than men.
- As discharged patients, women were less likely than men to have been prescribed appropriate medications.

Why Don't Women Take Better Care
of Themselves?

Women take more responsibility than men not only for their own health but for that of their families. They are more reliable than men about getting health checkups and taking medications. They are more willing to learn about their own health problems and those of family members. They are more comfortable discussing health problems with one another. They make better patients. So, while they are healthy, why don't women take better care of themselves?

"The problem is not lack of motivation," Dr. Julian Ford of the University of Connecticut Health Center told *The New York Times*. "It's competing motivations. Women tend to have too many priorities, and they find themselves pulled between them."

A woman has no time to call her own. Someone always needs something or something needs doing before she can think of herself. The more she does and the better she does it, the more others depend on her. She can only do so many things in a day. When she gets time to herself, she simply wants to take it easy.

"So much of my life is made up of doing what is required," women often say to Dr. Ford, "I really want to have something I enjoy."

In my practice, women patients seem to be more stressed than men. Many work outside the home. They wake up, get themselves ready for work, wake and dress the kids, get breakfast ready, and get the kids off to school. They then work a full day, pick up the kids from school, get home and fix dinner, help the kids with homework, clean up the kitchen, make cupcakes for the bake sale, get the kids ready for bed . . . you get the idea. Women seem to have less time to themselves than men. They show up in my office a "bundle of nerves," anxious and tense, with elevated blood pressure and elevated cholesterol. Cholesterol, by the way, is elevated by stress.

Clearly, women are not only affected differently by heart disease but must also be treated differently from men.

4. Why Knowing Your Cholesterol Level Isn't Enough

Joe, a 54-year-old bank executive, received a free annual medical checkup as a perk from his company. No health problems had been found in his previous checkups, and he didn't expect any from this year's either. The doctor examined him and said that everything looked normal. A week later, a nurse phoned to say the results of his lab tests had come in and they were all within normal ranges. She told him that his total cholesterol level was 199, which was below the recommended top level of 200. She also said that his general lab test results matched those of a much younger man. Flattered, Joe laughed and said he would see her again next year.

A week later, sitting at his desk at ten-thirty in the morning, Joe felt an ache in his left upper arm. He figured it was probably the way he had lain in bed. Twenty minutes later, he felt a pressure on his chest. It was like an invisible weight, so heavy he could hardly breathe.

"I don't like the way you look," a colleague said. "I'll call an ambulance."

"No, don't do that," Joe said. "It'll pass in a minute."

She called anyway. There was something about the way Joe looked that reminded her of her father the day he died suddenly. Joe told her later that her quick response had saved his life.

The paramedics put him on a stretcher while his fellow workers gathered around and looked at him with pity. Joe heard one tell another that he was having a heart attack.

"But my cholesterol is normal!" he called out.

The paramedics rushed him to the hospital. Their care on the way and the treatment he received in the emergency room enabled him to survive an acute myocardial infarction—medical terminology for a heart attack.

• • •

Approximately 1.1 million Americans a year have a heart attack. Half of them die. Of those who die, half do so within an hour of the attack's onset. It is thought that if they had received quick treatment, only 2 percent would have died. One in four Americans who have a fatal heart attack dies without medical treatment because they wait two or three hours before seeking help, even when they realize what is happening to them.

What happened to Joe happens, with minor variations, to people every day of the year. In fact, of the more than a million Americans who suffer a heart attack each year, at least half have total cholesterol levels that are normal or only slightly high.

But what about Joe's bad and good cholesterol levels?

Bad cholesterol (low-density lipoprotein, or LDL) participates in the buildup of plaque in the artery walls. Good cholesterol (high-density lipoprotein, or HDL) helps clear plaque out of our arteries. Joe's LDL blood level was a little over the desirable maximum, and his HDL level was a little under the desirable minimum. These weren't healthy levels, but neither were they a cause for immediate alarm. Although relatively small rises or falls in HDL or LDL blood levels can be important, no one's state of health strictly conforms to numbers.

Joe also did not have other heart attack risk factors.

High blood pressure? No.

Diabetes? No. His fasting glucose level was normal.

Smoker? No.

Some people with normal total cholesterol levels who have a heart attack, like Joe, have high LDL or low HDL. Or they smoke, have high blood pressure, or are diabetic. In their cases, a heart attack is explainable in other ways. But cases like Joe's mystify doctors. He had none of the usual risk factors and yet he had a heart attack.

Doctors don't like to be mystified by their patients. They are trained to rely on medical techniques in order to help people. When the medical techniques prove unreliable, they can make the doctors look incompetent or, worse, careless. This is why your doctor will probably hesitate to say that you don't need to worry about your heart as long as your lab test results are normal. Doctors know lab results don't necessarily tell the whole story.

Some Facts About Heart Disease in the United States

Bad News	Good News
Almost sixty million Americans— nearly 1 in every 4—have some kind of heart disease.	You cut your risk of heart disease in half by leading a physically active life or getting exercise.

Some Facts About Heart Disease in the United States *(continued)*

Bad News	*Good News*
Heart disease and stroke cause one of every two deaths—more deaths than all other diseases combined.	By losing as little as 5 to 10 percent of your body weight, you can substantially lower your risk of heart disease.
You are ten times more likely to die of heart disease than from a car accident, and thirty times more likely to die of heart disease than AIDS.	Eliminating just a few items of what you eat can sometimes help lower your blood fat levels.
Heart disease is equal opportunity, being the leading cause of death for both men and women in all ethnic groups.	If you stop smoking now, your risk of heart disease and stroke due to smoking will subside within five years.
The yearly cost of cardiovascular disease approaches $300 billion.	

New Explanation of Coronary Artery Disease

Most heart attacks result from coronary artery disease. The arteries feeding the heart muscle become blocked, the muscle cells are starved of oxygenated blood, and a heart attack follows. The first symptom of coronary artery disease may be chest pain, when blood flow though the coronary arteries becomes impeded by buildup of plaque on the interior artery wall. (Unfortunately, a heart attack is also likely to be the first "symptom," especially in men.) Much of the plaque that builds up on the artery wall consists of cholesterol and other fatty particles.

Buildup of plaque inside arteries is called "atherosclerosis." So long as doctors saw atherosclerosis solely as a matter of fatty particle buildup on the insides of arteries, in much the same way that gravel is deposited against a stream bank or sediment builds up inside an old pipe, it was natural for them to view cholesterol as the archenemy. The more cholesterol particles you had in your bloodstream, the greater the likelihood that cholesterol particles would be deposited in the form of plaque on your artery walls. Therefore, it was believed—and this continues to hold true—the higher your total cholesterol level, the higher your risk of coronary artery disease and a heart attack.

It's easy to understand how heart attack victims like Joe deeply concerned supporters of this simple, rational explanation of coronary artery disease. Many doctors, however, were well aware that the explanation could not be this simple. They themselves had seen or heard of too many cases like Joe's. They guessed that something else had to be involved. That something else proved to be inflammation.

Atherosclerosis is really an inflammatory disease of the delicate cells lining the interior artery wall. At first, this might not seem like anything startlingly new, but it changes the way we view plaque buildup. Plaque is no longer regarded as detritus—a collection of lifeless fatty particles, dead cells, and other rubbish. Instead, plaque is now known to be in large part living material, composed of modified white blood cells as well as fatty particles and dead cells. As part of their roles as agents of the immune system, these modified white blood cells secrete enzymes and other substances that affect the cells around them.

Inflammation is the body's cellular response to injury. Various kinds of white blood cells, activated by the immune system, travel through the bloodstream to the site of the injury. There they attack whatever is causing the injury. We looked at these white blood cells in Chapter 1. Suffice it to say that while warfare continues between the defender white blood cells and the invaders, inflammation persists.

What gives inflammation crucial importance is its role in the actual blockage of coronary arteries. The process of a heart attack is not caused by cholesterol-loaded plaque. At some stage in the inflammation process, the plaque ruptures and a blood clot forms at the rupture site. This blood clot on the surface of the ruptured plaque, rather than fatty particles, blocks the coronary artery and causes the heart attack. In other words, the heart attack is actually caused by the body's reaction to the ruptured plaque.

The levels of certain substances in the bloodstream rise during inflammation. Three of them are C-reactive protein, fibrinogen, and ferritin. Because doctors can use them to detect the presence of inflammation, these substances are known as "inflammatory markers."

New Indicators of Cardiac Risk

This new knowledge about coronary artery disease has resulted in some new lab tests for assessing heart attack risk and, given some existing tests, a new relevancy. For this book, I have selected six lab tests that cover risk areas beyond those covered by the regular blood lipid tests that you get in a health checkup. Three of the new tests are for inflammatory markers: C-reactive protein, fibrinogen, and ferritin. All six lab tests are presently available at reasonable prices at most doctors' offices and can all be performed on the blood sample you give for your regular lab tests. Most medical insurance plans cover these tests. But don't assume that you will receive them in a standard medical checkup. Be sure to specially request them. Also, make sure they are covered.

These are not the only tests possible. There are probably another twenty biological agents you could be tested for, but the problem with most of them is that they are not stable at room temperature and many need to be kept frozen. Under present circumstances, the tests would be very difficult to administer at a doctor's office and the lab results would be unreliable. Such tests are currently being studied under controlled conditions at research labs. Hopefully, they will become available at reasonable prices in the near future.

The seventh test, for calcium deposits in your arteries, requires a CT scan; it is expensive and not likely to be covered by your medical insurance company. Its one-of-a-kind results, however, make it worthwhile.

C-reactive Protein

The high-sensitivity C-reactive protein test is being hailed as the most accurate indicator of high heart attack risk available today. However, although a high C-reactive protein level indicates that inflammation is taking place somewhere in the body, the inflammation may not be in the coronary arteries and may have nothing to do with heart disease. Systemic inflammation, such as connective tissue diseases, may be responsible for the elevated C-protein. Local inflammation also needs to be considered, such as gum disease, prostatitis, urinary tract infections, and gastric inflammation.

All the same, inflammation elsewhere in the body seems to increase its likelihood in the coronary arteries as well.

Fibrinogen

Fibrinogen, a protein manufactured by the liver, is needed for blood to form a clot. On injury, fibrinogen is summoned into the bloodstream and converted to fibrin at the injury site. Fibrin forms into filaments, trapping blood cells and forming the clot. Fibrinogen is also known as "factor I." In the presence of inflammation, your blood level of fibrinogen rises sharply, acting as an inflammatory marker.

Homocysteine

Homocysteine is another indicator of cardiac risk. However, it remains a source of contention for doctors. While many people who have heart attacks have high homocysteine levels, no one has yet come up with a widely accepted explanation as to why. It's known that homocysteine itself is directly injurious to artery wall cells. If your doctor tries to dismiss your high homocysteine level because he or she doesn't understand how it works, mention aspirin. Doctors recommended aspirin for many years before they learned how it worked. It's the medical effect, not the scientific knowledge, that you need to care most about. On the other hand, instead of trying to convince your doctor, perhaps it's time you found a new one.

In spite of the fact that we know so little about how homocysteine operates, we know how to reduce its level in the blood. Over-the-counter, nonprescription supplements of folate and vitamins B-6 and B-12 achieve this, leading to the supposition that a high homocysteine level has something to do with a vitamin B deficiency. If only other heart issues were so easily solved!

Fasting Insulin

All the carbohydrates we eat, regardless of kind, are transformed into the sugar glucose in our blood. Our cells, assisted by the hormone insulin, use this blood sugar as fuel. With the help of insulin, the body stores much of the extra glucose as fat. An undetermined large number of Americans—perhaps one in four—inherit the genes for insulin resistance. "Insulin resistance" means that more insulin than normal is required to deal with a person's blood glucose. If you are insulin-resistant, you have a much greater chance of developing metabolic syndrome, which translates to a major risk of heart disease, as we saw in Chapter 2. A fasting insulin test is one way to detect if you have metabolic syndrome.

Insulin-resistant people are often obese and sedentary. Insulin resistance frequently leads to glucose intolerance and finally to type 2 diabetes. This kind of diabetes used to be referred to as "adult-onset diabetes." The fasting glucose test (in your regular battery of tests in a health checkup) checks you for diabetes. Don't confuse the fasting glucose test with the fasting insulin test.

Ferritin

An iron-protein complex, ferritin is one of the forms in which your body makes use of the mineral iron. We all know that people with too little iron in their blood are anemic. However, too much iron in the blood causes other problems, including some that affect the heart. People who have ferritin levels in the high normal range are at increased risk for heart disease. Ferritin is believed to promote the formation of free radicals, which raise the level of LDL and also cause damage to heart muscle and artery linings. It is also a marker of inflammation.

Lipoprotein(a)

Lipoprotein(a), or Lp(a), is an inflammatory marker that also plays an active role in atherosclerosis. It promotes the formation of blood clots and later slows their breaking up. In addition, Lp(a) helps cells transform themselves inside arterial plaque, increasing its size. When your Lp(a) level is high, as with fibrinogen, you have a greater chance of forming a clot on ruptured plaque and having a heart attack. With Lp(a) and fibrinogen, one test result confirms or contradicts the other. An Lp(a) test or fibrinogen test, or both, can indicate the presence of inflammation in cases where CRP fails to do so.

Calcium Heart Scan

A CT (computer tomography) scan of the heart and nearby arteries detects calcium deposits. Healthy arteries have no such deposits. Any calcium detected in your arteries is deposited inside plaque. The distribution and amount of the calcium permit experts to estimate the probability and extent of plaque in your coronary arteries.

Introduction to the Tests

This year, about 650,000 Americans will have their first heart attack. Many will have been careful about diet and exercise, and will never have had any cardiac symptoms. Many will die.

Quite a few will have had a fairly recent medical checkup in which their cholesterol level was normal or nearly so. I have great respect for cholesterol levels as an indicator for cardiac risk. When your cholesterol level is high, you need to take action to lower it. A good way to start is by increasing your activity, changing your diet, losing some weight, and learning relaxation techniques. If that doesn't work, you may need to take medication. I am not suggesting that these new tests should *replace* cholesterol level and other accepted tests for cardiac risk. A high cholesterol level is a cardiac danger signal that you cannot safely ignore. If some of your results from these new tests are elevated and your cholesterol level is also high, it may even be more important to treat your high cholesterol aggressively. However, simply because your cholesterol level is in the range presently defined as normal, you are not necessarily safe from a heart attack.

These seven new tests can provide a warning when your cholesterol level doesn't, or when other test results are borderline. If you have some reason to be concerned about your cardiac health—because of how you feel or how you live or because of your family medical history—these tests can possibly provide life-saving information.

Jeff was a borderline case. His cholesterol and triglyceride levels were a little above normal, as was his blood pressure. For a man of 41, he was overweight. He had a desk job, watched a lot of TV, and drank at least a six-pack of beer every evening.

A doctor had already told Jeff to lose weight, exercise, and come back again in three months, with the expectation that his lipid levels and blood pressure would drop if Jeff followed a healthier lifestyle. Jeff ignored his advice. The doctor referred him to me, I think, because he had a good diagnostic instinct. Because neither Jeff's lipid levels nor his blood pressure were threateningly high, I might have given him the same advice as his doctor had I not given him some of these new tests.

Fortunately for Jeff, I requested C-reactive protein and fibrinogen tests for him. Their results, in contrast to the other results, were alarmingly high. These test results indicated that Jeff had inflammation taking place in his body, very possibly in his coronary arteries. If this was where the inflammation was located, he had a possible increased risk of a heart attack.

On the other hand, if the results of Jeff's C-reactive protein and fibrinogen tests had come back in the normal range, I would have felt more reassured, as a physician, in sending him away for three months with good advice to change his lifestyle and no medication. So keep in mind that these new tests can bring good news and peace of mind.

These new tests cover areas of cardiac risk not covered by regular tests. Thus they can provide either an unexpected but timely warning or added assurance that all is well with your heart.

What These Seven Tests Can Do for You

In the chapters that are devoted to each test, we do the following:

- We look at the possible scores for each test and interpret the meanings of various levels.
- We consider what you need to do when your level is too high.
- We view the test results in conjunction with other tests, as well as with traditional risk factors for heart disease.

- We discuss the cautions necessary in interpreting test results.
- We mention physicians' disagreements or doubts.

When these tests confirm good news, they can give you genuine peace of mind about your cardiac condition. When these tests challenge what seem like good results from regular tests, they can warn you of unjustified or misplaced confidence. My advice is specific and realistic. By realistic, I mean that my expectations are modest. I always try to include a reward or enjoyment factor in my recommendations.

These seven tests give you increased monitoring power over an enlarged area of cardiac risk. I recommend them as a great improvement in watching over your own heart health and that of your loved ones.

Part II

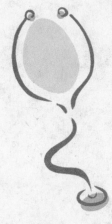

The Essential
New Tests

5. C-reactive Protein Test

C-REACTIVE PROTEIN TEST

What Is It?

A blood test to measure the level of C-reactive protein

Test Results

Above 3 milligrams per liter (mg/L) of blood	High risk
1–3 mg/L	Borderline risk
Below 1 mg/L	Low risk

Cost Without Medical Insurance

About $20

Increases CRP Levels

Chronic infections (gum disease, bronchitis)

Increases CRP Levels (continued)

Chronic inflammation (rheumatoid arthritis)

Diabetes

High blood pressure

Hormone replacement therapy

Low HDL level and high triglyceride level

Metabolic syndrome

Smoking

Lowers CRP levels

Abciximab

Aspirin

Clopidogrel

Fibrates

Gemfibrozil

Moderate alcohol consumption

Moderate exercise

Niacin

Statins

Thiazolidinedione diabetes drugs

Weight loss

C-reactive protein (CRP) is a marker of inflammation and predictor of heart attacks, strokes, peripheral artery disease, and sudden cardiac death. It is made in the liver. While not normally found in the blood, it quickly appears after inflammation, bacterial or fungal infections, or injury. It quickly disappears from the blood when its trigger has been eliminated.

CRP is independent of the usual cardiac risk factors considered by doctors, such as age, smoking, cholesterol level, blood pressure, and diabetes. It works as a predictor equally well in men and women, smokers and nonsmokers, the elderly and middle-aged, diabetics and nondiabetics, and people of various races.

Some doctors believe that one CRP test is sufficient. To avoid the chance of a misleading result from a passing minor infection, most doctors recommend two tests approximately two weeks apart, with the lower result being taken as the level of cardiac risk. Because major infections or illness can result in alarmingly high but temporary CRP levels, doctors usually schedule another test for a later date if someone's CRP level is 10 mg/L or above. In rare cases, high CRP levels are caused by lupus, inflammatory bowel disease, or endocarditis. Someone suffering from one of these conditions usually also has a high result from an erythrocyte sedimentation rate test, another nonspecific marker of inflammation.

You don't need to fast for your CRP test, because the level is not affected by what you eat or the time of day the test is administered. Your CRP level is likely to be steady over an extended period. If your result is normal, your doctor is likely to schedule your next CRP test with your next cholesterol test, usually once a year. No benefit has been shown from a series of more frequent CRP tests.

Make sure that you receive a high-sensitivity CRP test, often designated "hs-CRP," by asking your doctor for it specifically. The older kinds of CRP tests are not sufficiently sensitive to detect the levels required for prediction of heart attack risk.

Why C-reactive Protein?

C-reactive protein is not the only inflammatory marker that can predict heart attacks and strokes. Tests that measure cytokine activity and cellular adhesion are good predictors. So too are tests that measure immunologic function, such as tests for interleukin-6, intercellular adhesion molecule-1, macrophage inhibitory cytokine-1, and soluble CD40 ligand. However, either these tests are too difficult to perform on a regular basis in a doctor's office or the substance involved is too unstable under normal conditions. C-reactive protein is reliable and convenient. CRP levels can be accurately tested in either fresh or frozen blood samples.

Initially doctors were concerned that a high CRP level caused by inflammation outside the cardiovascular system might raise a false alarm. "The bottom line is that we now understand that inflammation from virtually any cause in fact leads to markedly elevated cardiac risk," Dr. Paul Ridker of the Harvard Medical School told *The Wall Street Journal*. In other words, if your CRP is high for any reason, you have reason to be concerned.

Missing a night's sleep or undergoing short-term sleep deprivation causes the CRP level to rise, according to Dr. H. K. Meier-Ewert and colleagues at the Lahey Clinic Medical Center in Boston. They noted that lack of sleep and short-term sleep duration are known to be linked to cardiovascular disease, and that insufficient sleep may trigger inflammation processes inside arteries.

In Wales, bodybuilders taking anabolic androgenic steroids had significantly higher CRP levels and correspondingly higher cardiovascular risks.

Besides being a marker of inflammation, CRP plays a direct role in atherosclerosis by secreting substances that help bind adhesion molecules to the artery wall and that promote LDL uptake by macrophages in the artery wall.

Health Organization
Recommendations

"The horse is out of the barn," said Dr. Thomas Pearson, senior associate dean for clinical research at the University of Rochester School of Medicine and Dentistry in New York State. He was talking about the recommendation in favor of testing for CRP levels by two prominent health organizations, the first such recommendation in twenty years. In January 2003, the American Heart Association and the Centers for Disease Control and Prevention recommended the test and issued guidelines for it. The American Heart Association reports that a high CRP level raises your risk of a heart attack two to five times.

The guidelines suggest that people with a moderate risk of heart disease should take the test. About 40 percent of adult Americans have a "moderate" risk of heart disease, according to Dr. Sidney C. Smith Jr., a cardiologist at the University of North Carolina at Chapel Hill (see Chapter 12 for cardiac risk levels). But even when other tests tell you that you have only moderate risk, you may be at higher risk if you have inflammation in your arteries. The CRP test detects such inflammation.

According to the guidelines, people at very low risk of a heart attack don't need to take a CRP test. Neither do people who have already been diagnosed with heart disease or diabetes, because they are probably already taking a statin. You need to take the test, the guidelines say, if you are in the gray zone—if you are aged 50 or more and have one or more of the following risk factors: you smoke or you have high blood pressure, a high cholesterol level, or a family history of heart disease. Already doctors are using the CRP test for a much wider selection of patients, which was what Dr. Pearson meant by saying that the horse was out of the barn. Simply put,

CRP is a predictor of cardiac events. In my view, anyone who needs to take a cholesterol test also needs to take a CRP test.

CRP Level and LDL Cholesterol Level

Your CRP level is a better predictor of cardiovascular disease than your LDL cholesterol level, according to Dr. Paul M. Ridker and colleagues at Brigham and Women's Hospital. Their study was based on blood samples from nearly 28,000 seemingly healthy women, whose health was then followed for eight years. This is by far the largest study of the connection between CRP and cardiovascular disease. The women's CRP levels were directly related to heart attacks, strokes, and other kinds of cardiovascular disease, and were a better predictor of them than their LDL levels. Women with the highest CRP levels were twice as likely as those with a high LDL level to have a heart attack or stroke or to die from heart disease. Women with a high CRP and low LDL were at higher risk than women with a low CRP and high LDL. Many doctors today are not aware of this risk differential.

According to one estimate, 25 to 30 million Americans have normal or low LDL levels but high CRP levels, and therefore a high cardiovascular risk level. Most don't know this, and this risk to their lives is likely to be overlooked by many of their doctors. So even when your LDL is below 130, if your CRP is above 3 mg/L, you are at high risk.

"Across the board, CRP proved to be a better predictor than LDL," Dr. Ridker claimed. He pointed out that CRP levels may be rising over a period of twenty-five to thirty years in people before they have a heart attack or stroke. Dr. Ridker also said that people who lower their LDL levels with statins can be deceived into thinking they don't have to diet or exercise anymore. If their CRP levels remain high, so does their cardio-vascular risk.

Dr. Ridker's study was part of the Women's Health Study, which began early in the 1990s. Its original purpose was to see whether aspirin and vitamin E helped prevent heart attacks in healthy women over the age of 45. Dr. Ridker and his colleagues measured the LDL and CRP levels in blood samples and then checked to see how they influenced the women's cardiovascular health later on. Of the nearly 28,000 women, 571 had a heart attack, stroke, or heart-related surgery. Dr. Ridker found that almost 4 out of 5 cardiac events happened to women whose LDL was under 160 (130 to 160 is the normal range). Almost half the cardiac events occurred in women whose LDL was under 130 (in the desirable or better than normal range).

Here's what you need to consider if you have a high CRP:

- *LDL above 160 and high CRP:* You need drug therapy and a healthier lifestyle without delay.
- *LDL 130–160 and high CRP:* You need to comply care-fully with the therapy your doctor recommends and be sure to diet and exercise.
- *LDL below 130 and high CRP:* Don't be deceived by your LDL. Your high CRP level indicates that your cardiac risk is high. You need to comply with your doctor's therapy and watch your lifestyle. You may also be at risk for meta-bolic syndrome and should have a fasting glucose test. A large-scale study is under way to see if people with these levels should take statins.

If your CRP continues to remain elevated, it may be benefi-cial to lower your LDL to below 80, especially if you already have coronary artery disease.

A later study by Dr. Ridker showed that for people taking statins, those whose CRP levels were lowered had better health outcomes than those whose CRP levels were not, regardless of their LDL levels. Another recent study found that the slowing of atherosclerosis with intensive statin therapy corresponded to a drop in CRP level.

• PENNY'S STORY •

When all your lab results are more or less normal, except your CRP, the next step can be a close call. Penny's CRP was 3.5 after a second test, and her cholesterol was mildly elevated, only 242. Her LDL was 132. But she also had high blood pressure and she smoked. Her doctor was reluctant to put her, at the age of 53, on a statin—usually a lifelong medication. She sent Penny to see me. Other than what her doctor had already diagnosed, I could find nothing wrong. I put her on a statin, which brought her CRP level down to 1.5 in two months, which is about the best result I have seen. On my instructions, Penny refilled the prescription twice, then went three months without the statin, and came back to be tested again. Her CRP was about the same. I did not renew the prescription.

On checkups with her regular doctor since that time, her CRP level has remained in that range and she has developed no other cardiac risk factors. This is not bad for a smoker with high blood pressure. What would have happened if her CRP level hadn't been reduced? I don't know. I can't even be sure the inflammation that caused her elevated CRP level was in an artery.

While we now have the ability to lower LDL levels with statins, I'm finding an increasing number of cognitive problems in people taking this type of medication. (For more on this area of concern, see "How Safe Are Statins?" in Chapter 12.)

• • •

CRP Performance as a Predictor

People with the highest levels of CRP have twice the risk of heart attacks as people with the lowest levels, according to an analysis of fourteen long-term studies by Dr. Mary S. Beattie and colleagues at the University of California at San Francisco. Dr. Beattie showed that among people with coronary disease, those with the highest CRP levels were about four times more likely to show evidence of impaired blood flow during a treadmill test.

In the ongoing Physicians' Health Study of 22,000 men, 97 apparently healthy participants died suddenly of heart disease, according to Dr. Christine M. Albert and colleagues at Brigham and Women's Hospital in Boston. Over seventeen years of observation in the study, the only thing they had in common that could have predicted their deaths was an elevated CRP level.

Women on hormone replacement therapy (HRT) were warned of a rise in CRP level, but it has turned out that their slightly higher CRP levels are not sufficiently altered to be significant.

CRP levels only minimally rise or fall with cholesterol levels, and there is no way to estimate your CRP level from your cholesterol level.

Normal CRP ranges have yet to be established for young adults and children. Discovering high CRP levels in their offspring could provide parents with an early warning that lifestyle changes need to be made to ensure the health of their children.

When CRP Fails

CRP's record as a predictor of heart trouble is not perfect, according to Dr. Peter Libby and colleagues at the Harvard Medical

School. When people have unstable angina and a major heart attack risk, about 70 percent of them have a high CRP. But when their angina is stable or variant and their risk high, only about 20 percent have a high CRP. This could lead them to a sense of false security about their heart condition.

Not everyone with unstable angina and elevated CRP has a heart attack. But practically everyone who complains of unstable angina before having a heart attack is found to have elevated CRP on admission to the hospital.

When a CRP test fails to predict heart trouble about to occur, a fibrinogen test can take its place. It was reported at an American Heart Association conference in 2001 that for people with cardiovascular disease, fibrinogen, but not CRP, proved to be a reliable predictor of recurring cardiovascular events.

CRP as a Predictor of Metabolic Syndrome and Diabetes

Inflammation, but not necessarily an elevated LDL cholesterol level, is involved in the health problems of the metabolic syndrome (syndrome X). These include high triglyceride levels, obesity, high blood pressure, and high blood sugar, as well as associated conditions often missed by doctors, such as insulin resistance, clotting problems, and dysfunction of artery linings. Thus, a high CRP level can be a warning of metabolic syndrome processes, as well as of atherosclerosis.

Inflammation, atherosclerosis, and type 2 diabetes are tightly interrelated disorders of the immune system. According to different studies by A. D. Pradhan and Paul M. Ridker, a high CRP level may also be an indicator of a risk for diabetes.

Lowering Your CRP Level

Weight loss, a healthy diet, exercise, and stopping smoking reduce your CRP level.

The cholesterol-lowering drugs called statins can lower your CRP level by 15 to 25 percent in as little as six weeks. Although your LDL cholesterol level is always lowered by statins, you can't assume that your CRP level has gone down just because your LDL level has. Statins don't lower everybody's CRP levels. To what extent this happens is presently being investigated. Generally speaking, however, people with high CRP levels do very well on statins in reducing those levels and their overall cardiac risk.

How to Reduce Inflammation

- Eat foods rich in omega-3 fatty acids. Eat fatty, coldwater fish such as salmon, trout, tuna, mackerel, sardines, or herring at least once a week. Alternatively, take a fish oil supplement that has been tested for mercury contamination.
- Brush your teeth regularly and have your teeth cleaned at your dentist's office at least once a year. This helps prevent the development of dental plaque and growth of bacteria responsible for inflammatory gum disease.
- Trim your waistline. Body fat at waist level helps elevate your CRP level.
- Moderate exercise stimulates your muscles and bodily functions.
- Add some flaxseed to your food.
- Add some anti-inflammatory spices to your food, such as ginger, turmeric, and cumin.

6. Fibrinogen Test

FIBRINOGEN TEST

What Is It?

A blood test to measure the level of the protein fibrinogen

Test Results

Above 460 milligrams per deciliter (mg/dL) of blood	High risk
300–460 mg/dL	Borderline high risk (though often regarded within normal range)
150–299 mg/dL	Normal

Cost Without Medical Insurance

About $100

Increases Fibrinogen Level

Estrogen supplements
High animal-protein diet
High saturated-fat diet
High homocysteine level
Infections

Lack of exercise
Oral contraceptives
Smoking
Vitamin B deficiency

Lowers Fibrinogen Level

Anabolic steroids
Androgens
Blood transfusions (banked blood
   has no fibrinogen)
Bone marrow lesions
Congenital lack of, low, or abnormal
   fibrinogen
Curcumin (spice)
Exercise
Ginger root (spice)
Liver disease

Lung disease
Malnourishment
Obstetric complications
Omega-3 fatty acids
Phenobarbital
Prostate cancer
Some bleeding disorders
Streptokinase
Turmeric (spice)
Urokinase
Valproic acid

I f you are actively bleeding or have an acute infection or illness, postpone your fibrinogen test until your condition has cleared. Also, don't have a test within four weeks of having received a blood transfusion.

One of the amazing things about a healthy body is the ability of the blood to clot just the right amount, at the right time and right place, to stop bleeding from a wound. If clots form too easily, a person could have a stroke. On the other hand, if clots do not form in time, a person could bleed to death. The body makes substances that promote clot formation, and other substances that break up clots. The balance between these substances controls clot formation and breakup.

Fibrinogen, a protein made by the liver, is best known for its role as a blood clotting or coagulation factor—it is known as "factor I." When your body detects an injury, fibrinogen production by your liver can increase fourfold. Fibrinogen and blood platelets are sent through your blood to the injury site. At the wound, these platelets stick to one another, helped by fibrinogen and lipoprotein(a). They are bound together by fibrin (derived from fibrinogen), forming a clot to seal off the wound and prevent further loss of blood. High levels of fibrinogen in the blood permit the making of large clots.

If you had a cut on your hand that permitted external bleeding, or damage to a blood vessel that allowed internal bleeding, clotting would be a beneficial reaction. But if you have inflamed plaque in a coronary artery that is in danger of rupturing, the last thing you need in your blood is a large quantity of a substance that promotes clotting. The higher the fibrinogen level and the blood's clot-forming capability, the greater the likelihood of a clot forming on ruptured plaque and causing a heart attack.

Besides adhering to one another, platelets at an injury site in an artery can secrete substances that cause the artery walls to contract. Fibrinogen also has the power to do this. This constriction of an artery increases the chances of a clot blocking blood flow.

Foods rich in saturated fat and animal protein help raise the blood level of fibrinogen. One of the ways that hormone replacement therapy (HRT) elevates the risk of heart disease in women is through raising their fibrinogen levels and making clots within their arteries more likely. Cancers of the stomach, breast, or kidney and inflammatory disorders, such as rheumatoid arthritis and acute pneumonia, also cause high fibrinogen levels.

Foods rich in omega-3 fatty acids, such as salmon, may decrease your fibrinogen level.

• A BASEBALL PLAYER •

I was asked to see a retired professional baseball player who had suffered a heart attack. The 48-year-old ex-player's career now involved promoting several commercial products, and his agent was trying to downplay his heart attack to "exhaustion" status.

"His cholesterol is normal," the agent informed me.

This was true. His LDL was 105. He had no diabetes, high blood pressure, or family history of heart disease, and he didn't smoke. But he had high fibrinogen and C-reactive protein, and very high homocysteine.

I prescribed a statin and high-dose vitamin B-complex supplements. They brought his fibrinogen and homocysteine levels down to a normal range and his LDL down to 70. He recovered from his "exhaustion." He went through cardiac rehabilitation and made some lifestyle changes, including yoga, meditation, and a relaxation technique. Eventually he was able to discontinue taking statins, but continued taking B-complex vitamins. His fibrinogen and C-reactive protein have remained low.

• • •

How a High Fibrinogen Level Can Affect You

Moderate exercise and vitamin B supplements are the simple and inexpensive solutions to a high fibrinogen level. A study of 3,800 British men aged 60 through 79 who exercised regularly showed they had reduced levels of fibrinogen and CRP. The researchers, led by Dr. S. G. Wannamethee, also found that their blood was less viscous. Less viscous blood flows more freely through arteries and is less likely to adhere to artery walls.

In the Scottish Heart Healthy Study, fibrinogen levels and blood viscosity were followed for thirteen years in 1,238 men and women aged 25 to 64. A high fibrinogen level was found to be the chief cause of higher blood viscosity that resulted in death.

The risk of a heart attack or stroke almost doubles with very high fibrinogen levels, according to Dr. B. R. Jaeger and Dr. C. A. Labarrere of the Munich University Clinic in Germany. For them, fibrinogen worked as a cardiac predictor equally well in men and women, young and old, and for first-time and repeat heart attacks or strokes. Drug therapy with the prescription medications known as "fibrates" resulted in moderate lowering of fibrinogen and cholesterol levels. This worked well as a preventive strategy against repeat heart attacks and strokes.

Some researchers worked with blood vessels in the limbs, called the "peripheral vascular system." In peripheral arteries, fibrinogen is more important than cholesterol, triglycerides, C-reactive protein, and immunoglobulins in maintaining the adhesiveness and aggregation of red blood cells, according to Dr. V. Schechner and colleagues at Tel Aviv Sourasky Medical Center in Israel. In people with peripheral artery disease being treated at the University of Vienna Medical School in Austria, those with the highest fibrinogen levels were more likely to have a poor outcome, particularly fatal cardiovascular complications.

Margarine and Fibrinogen

Margarine containing plant sterols or stanols, as well as margarine enriched with omega-6 fatty acids, is known to reduce LDL levels. These margarines were tested on forty-two healthy male students, with an average age of 23, at the National Institute of Food and Nutrition in Warsaw, Poland. How such margarines affect fibrinogen levels and platelet activity is unknown.

Margarine with plant sterols caused an 11 percent drop in LDL. Margarine enriched with omega-6 fatty acids caused a 6 percent reduction of LDL and a 3 percent rise in HDL. Both margarines caused a slight rise in fibrinogen levels without exceeding the normal range. With both margarines, blood platelets grew less sticky and took a longer time to gather together, thereby becoming less prone to forming a clot.

The slight rise in fibrinogen level was not enough to offset the beneficial effects of both margarines on LDL and platelets, and of the omega-6 margarine on HDL.

If you are already using these margarines to lower cholesterol, you may want to consider products that combine the plant sterols with omega-3 fats rather than margarine. Margarine is high in trans fats, which appear to be problematic in themselves.

Do You Get Enough Vitamin B?

You can lower your fibrinogen level through moderate exercise and B-complex vitamins. (See "Do Vitamin B Supplements Work?" in Chapter 7.) The B-complex vitamins involved in lowering fibrinogen levels are the same as for lowering homocysteine levels: folic acid, B-6, and B-12.

The B-complex vitamins help the body convert carbohydrates into blood sugar to be used for energy. Natural foods are the best sources for vitamins, because foods probably include combinations of micronutrients that are missing from manufactured vitamin supplements. The presence of these miniscule quantities of unknown or little-known nutrients may be hugely important. Such micronutrients are also often lost in processed foods.

Many Americans have a vitamin B deficiency because of imbalances in their daily diets. It's not that easy to get all the vitamin B you need from readily available foods. The following natural food sources for folic acid, B-6, and B-12 can give you an idea of whether you derive sufficient vitamin B from the foods you eat regularly or whether you should take supplements.

Folic Acid from Foods

Folic acid at levels sufficient to satisfy your daily requirements is found in the following foods: barley, beans, beef, bran, brewer's yeast, brown rice, cheese, chicken, dates, green leafy vegetables, lamb, lentils, liver, milk, oranges, organ meats, peas, pork, root vegetables, salmon, tuna, wheat germ, whole wheat, and yeast. Because the concentrations of nutrients vary widely in unpackaged foods, it is difficult to match amounts of food to amounts of nutrient without testing a particular food sample.

You may need more than the normal daily requirement of folic acid (400 micrograms) if you take oral contraceptives. People with a convulsive disorder or hormone-related cancer should not take high doses of folic acid for an extended period.

B-6 from Foods

Vitamin B-6 (pyridoxine) exists in small amounts in all foods. The following foods contain relatively large amounts: brewer's yeast, carrots, chicken, eggs, fish, meat, peas, spinach, sunflower seeds, walnuts, and wheat germ. Lesser but still generous amounts of B-6 exist in avocado, bananas, beans, blackstrap molasses, brown rice, cabbage, cantaloupe, and whole grains.

If you take antidepressants, estrogen, or oral contraceptives, you may need extra amounts of vitamin B-6.

B-12 from Foods

Vitamin B-12 (cyanocobalamin) is not found in vegetables. Thus vegetarians are most likely to be deficient in this vitamin. People with digestive problems and the elderly also often have a vitamin B-12 deficiency. Obtainable only from animal sources, B-12 is found most plentifully in blue cheese, cheese, clams, eggs, herring, kidney, liver, mackerel, milk, seafood, and tofu.

You may need extra B-12 if you take potassium supplements, anticoagulants, or drugs for gout. The metabolic roles of folic acid and vitamin B-12 are intertwined, and a deficit in one can cause a deficit in the other.

Taking Vitamin B Supplements

If you have a high fibrinogen level and think that you may not get enough folic acid, B-6, and B-12 from foods, take vitamin B supplements. The recommended daily allowance (RDA) for folic acid is 400 micrograms; for B-6, 2 milligrams; and for B-12, 6 micrograms. I recommend taking at least double the RDA for each daily. You can do this most conveniently and economically by taking B-complex pills rather than separate pills for each. Read the label carefully to see which B supplements are included and in what quantities.

Other Therapeutic Approaches

Quitting smoking causes a reduction in fibrinogen level of about 150 mg/L. Starting to smoke causes an equal rise in the level. The fibrinogen level rises or falls according to the number of ciga-rettes smoked.

Apart from smokers, those most likely to have high fibrogen levels are people with diabetes, high blood pressure, obesity, or sedentary lifestyles. Any improvement in these conditions has the potential of lowering the fibrinogen level.

Statins and aspirin don't lower fibrinogen levels. Fibrates and niacin do.

7. Homocysteine Test

HOMOCYSTEINE TEST

What Is It?

A blood test to measure the level of the amino acid homocysteine

Test Results

Above 14 micromoles per liter (µmol/L) of blood	High risk
1–14 µmol/L	Borderline high risk
Below 10 µmol/L	Normal

Cost Without Medical Insurance

About $200

Increases Homocysteine Level

Coffee	
Estrogen deficiency	Organ transplants

Increases Homocysteine Level (continued)

High animal-protein diet	Smoking
	Thyroid hormone deficiencies
Hostility and stress	Vitamin B deficiencies (folic acid, B-6, B-12)
Kidney failure	

Lowers Homocysteine Level

Vitamin B

Exercise

Not all doctors agree on what homocysteine does and how important it is in cardiovascular disease. Many people with heart disease have high homocysteine levels—there's no argument about that. But is homocysteine simply a marker of inflammation or is it actually involved in the process of atherosclerosis? In my experience, I have good reason to believe that homocysteine is both. It certainly appears to be a predictor of heart attacks—and that's what concerns us here.

In 1969, Dr. Kilmer S. McCully, at Harvard Medical School and the Massachusetts General Hospital, was the first to link homocysteine levels to arterial disease. He noted that children with the inherited disorder homocystinuria had extremely high homocysteine levels, developed severe arterial disease, and died young. His work was not accepted by the medical establishment, and he subsequently lost his research funding and teaching positions. Only in recent years, with increasingly widespread recognition of homocysteine as a risk factor for heart disease, has Dr. McCully's pioneering work received respect.

Evidence has been accumulating of homocysteine's role in arterial disease. However, not only did it not have a role to play in the cholesterol explanation of heart disease, the big drug companies had no incentive to fund research in homocysteine. Unlike those for cholesterol, its remedies—taking vitamin B supplements and eating less animal protein—cannot be patented.

Homocysteine, at a high concentration in the bloodstream, is now believed to damage the delicate cells lining arteries and stimulate the growth of smooth muscle cells. This helps to trigger the process of atherosclerosis. Homocysteine is also believed to contribute to blood clot formation on ruptured plaque. In addition, it generates free radicals that oxidize LDL particles in the artery wall, enlarging plaque.

When methionine, an amino acid, is not completely converted to cysteine in the body, homocysteine remains as an intermediate product. The conversion is not completed for lack of a vitamin B–dependent enzyme, which is why B-complex deficiencies are held responsible for high homocysteine levels.

In the Physicians' Health Study, those among the 15,000 participating doctors who had a homocysteine level of 15 or more were three times as likely to have a heart attack as those with lower levels. Those with a level of 12 were twice as likely to have a heart attack, according to the research of Dr. Meir Stampfer and colleagues at the Harvard School of Public Health.

Similarities Between Homocysteine and Cholesterol

Homocysteine, although it is a protein, has much in common with the lipid cholesterol. The blood levels of both tend to rise with age. Men usually have higher levels of both, until women reach menopause, when levels become equal. In a number of reports, researchers have found homocysteine equal to high cholesterol levels and cigarette smoking as a cardiovascular risk factor. One analysis equated the risk of a rise in 5 μmol/L in homocysteine level with a rise of 20 in total cholesterol level.

Like cholesterol, homocysteine interacts with the multiple risk factors of diabetics to increase overall risk. Dutch researchers found that for every rise of 5 in homocysteine level, diabetics were more than three times as likely to die from any cause over a five-year period than nondiabetics with the same level of homocysteine.

Homocysteine as a Source of Free Radicals

Homocysteine acts as a source of free radicals in the artery wall. A free radical can be thought of as half a molecule looking for the other half. Once the free radical meets an agreeable partner, it forms a whole molecule. That molecule may be beneficial or harmful. When plenty of free radicals are in circulation, chances are increased that harmful molecules will be formed.

Oxidants are the kind of free radical generated by homocysteine in the artery wall. When something combines with an oxygen free radical, it becomes oxidized. In a familiar example, when iron is oxidized it rusts. We know that LDL particles that have entered the artery wall become oxidized, but accounts differ on what happens exactly. By some accounts, LDL and homocysteine particles that have invaded the artery wall are engulfed by macrophages and monocytes, the white blood cells that come to fight the invaders. Free radicals may help change the successful attackers into foam cells through oxidation, and thus build plaque. More basically, free radicals may simply cause LDL particles to decay inside the artery wall through oxidation, in the same way that contact with oxygen causes food to decay. Because oxygen is involved in all biochemical processes, the possibilities are endless.

White blood cells, lipid particles, and homocysteine are a deadly combination for the heart when all three are plentiful in the bloodstream. White blood cells are plentiful when the body detects inflammation. Lipid particles are plentiful when we eat high-fat diets, are overweight, and don't get enough exercise. Insufficient B-complex vitamins may be responsible for homocysteine concentrations. Although details still need to be worked out, nothing here is a mystery. A high level of homocysteine is dangerous to your heart. Homocysteine is several times more dangerous when combined with high LDL. Additionally, it collaborates with other cardiac risk factors. No matter how you look at it, a high homocysteine level is clearly a risk to cardiac health.

Vulnerable to Homocysteine

High homocysteine blood levels run in families. In families with a severe inherited condition, atherosclerosis develops in childhood and family members often have a heart attack by the age of 20. In the Third National Health and Nutrition Examination Survey, boys and girls aged 12 to 16 years with high homocysteine levels had parents with a history of high blood pressure or stroke before age 50. Adolescent boys with high homocysteine levels also tended to have high systolic blood pressure.

Studies of homocysteine usually have involved men. Of the few studies on women, none have lasted longer than thirteen years. Recently, with this in mind, Swedish doctors looked at data from the Population Study of Women in Gothenburg, which was begun during 1968–1969. For a follow-up period of twenty-four years, they found that, as in men, a high homocysteine level is an independent risk factor for heart attack in middle-aged women. In particular, high homocysteine was associated with women's deaths from heart attacks.

People with thyroid deficiencies, chronic kidney failure, or organ transplants are at risk for high homocysteine levels. If they smoke or have other cardiac risk factors, even a moderately elevated homocysteine level significantly increases their risk.

Stress can raise your homocysteine level. Even low levels of stress can produce a temporary effect. Some stress-reduction techniques may contribute to the health of our hearts through lowering homocysteine levels.

Pregnancy Complications

In pregnant women, elevated blood levels of homocysteine can be responsible for high blood pressure, early miscarriage, premature birth, very low birth weight, and birth defects. A woman who takes folic acid supplements during the first three weeks of pregnancy greatly lowers the risk of having a child with a spinal deformity. As a result of this finding, in 1998 the Food and Drug Administration ordered all flour and grain products to be fortified with folic acid. This may have reduced the homocysteine levels of Americans by 10 percent.

Aging Effects

Doctors have noticed for some time that a vitamin B deficiency can be responsible for cognitive decline in elderly people.

Vitamin B supplements—folic acid, B-6, and B-12—can improve impaired cognitive performance. Damage may be caused to small arteries in the brain by high homocysteine levels, according to Dr. Jacob Selhub and colleagues at the U.S. Department of Agriculture Human Nutrition Research Center on Aging at Tufts University in Boston.

After taking a blood sample, researchers followed the health of thirty nuns in a convent who ate the same food, lived the same simple life, and lived to the ages of 78 to 101. Those whose blood sample had a low level of folic acid were more likely to develop atrophy of the cerebral cortex. The lower the blood level of folic acid, the greater the atrophy, according to Dr. David A. Snowdon and colleagues at the University of Kentucky College of Medicine in Lexington.

Osteoporosis and presbyopia (difficulty in reading small print as we age) in the elderly have been linked to moderately high homocysteine levels by Dr. Carlos L. Krumdieck and Dr. Charles W. Prince at the University of Alabama School of Medicine in Birmingham. They told *The New York Times* that such "diseases of old age may have gone unrecognized because we are conditioned to accept them as inescapable consequences of growing old."

Diabetes and High Homocysteine Levels

Diabetics are twice as likely to be affected by heart disease as nondiabetics. In fact, more than three-quarters of all Americans with type 2 diabetes die from cardiovascular complications. A high homocysteine level has been shown to be an even greater risk factor for heart disease in diabetics than nondiabetics, making it all the more important that people with type 2 diabetes do something about high homocysteine.

Plaque buildup in arteries leading to the limbs, called "peripheral vascular disease," is a major complication of diabetes and cause of death. Elevated homocysteine is a stronger risk factor for peripheral vascular disease in diabetics than nondiabetics.

People with diabetes have two to four times greater risk of stroke. They also have a higher recurrence rate and poorer outcome. High homocysteine is a greater risk factor for stroke in diabetics than nondiabetics and an independent predictor of recurrent stroke.

About 70 percent of diabetics have high blood pressure. As homocysteine levels rise, so does the risk for high blood pressure. Homocysteine may start a chain of reactions that lead to high blood pressure.

Diabetes-induced kidney disease, called "diabetic nephropathy," creates the most frequent need for dialysis in the United States. In people with chronic kidney failure, high homocysteine is the most frequently found cardiovascular risk factor. The prevalence and severity of kidney failure in diabetics is associated with their homocysteine levels.

"Diabetic retinopathy" is an eye disease in which high glucose levels damage small eye arteries, causing blurred vision or blindness. It's the leading cause of adult blindness in the United States, with up to 24,000 new cases each year. High homocysteine levels are associated with the prevalence and severity of retinopathy in people with type 2 diabetes.

Up to 70 percent of diabetics have diabetes-induced nerve damage, called "diabetic neuropathy." High glucose impairs the ability of nerves to send messages, which can result in pain or numbness in hands, feet, and legs. High homocysteine levels are associated with the prevalence and severity of diabetic neuropathy in people with type 2 diabetes. An increase in homocysteine level of 5 micromoles can increase the risk for diabetic neuropathy by more than 150 percent.

Health Problems Linked to High Homocysteine Levels

Birth defects

Clots in veins

Dementia

Early miscarriage

Heart attack

High blood pressure during
  pregnancy

Osteoporosis

Premature birth

Presbyopia

Stroke

Very low birth weight

• KEVIN'S STORY •

The doctor phoned Kevin a week after his checkup to say his lab results were in and they were all within normal ranges. Kevin wondered why the doctor himself was calling.

"Your lipids are very good," the doctor said. "But you have high blood pressure and you smoke."

"Only a pack a day," Kevin said.

"Smoke five or smoke twenty," the doctor snapped, "the effects are the same. As for your blood pressure, it's still way too high, in spite of the medications you are taking for it."

"I've been tense lately," Kevin said. "And that day, getting to your office, I had a terrible time in traffic."

"Maybe," the doctor said, with doubt in his voice. "But I want you to see a cardiologist."

I heard all this when Kevin came to see me. Fifty years old, he was an ex-truck driver who now sold tractor trailers. He looked the part—big, tough, and significantly overweight at 275 pounds. He was solid and not flabby. His blood pressure remained at the same high level, and he had not quit smoking. His lab results came in a few days later. His cholesterol was good. At 17.3, his homocysteine level, which had not been tested before, was high. I had him return to my office to warn him of the particularly high heart attack risk posed by smoking, high blood pressure, and high homocysteine. The combination of these three risk factors, for some reason, is deadly. Kevin hardly listened to what I said.

If his cholesterol level had been high, he might have listened, but he didn't pay attention to something he had never heard of before, like homocysteine. It required much persuasion on my part to get him on a modified diet. This modified diet cut back on both saturated fats and carbohydrates such as starches, simple sugars, and refined grains, as well as foods with a high glycemic index. He also took to walking about forty-five minutes each day. The diet and moderate exercise lowered his homocysteine level and, as he lost weight, his blood pressure also came down. First, he lost a lot of fluid, and then he lost fat. After four months, he had lost thirty pounds. And he went from taking three medications for high blood pressure down to one. But he continued to smoke.

I'm not the kind of doctor who tells patients to quit smoking or don't bother coming back to see me because if they don't, then there's nothing I can do for them. I doubt if there are any smokers in the United States who have not heard they should quit for the sake of their health. I see my job as offering them assistance and providing them with the resources to enable them to stop. Whether they do so is up to them.

My general approach to healing is providing people with the resources so that they can do it themselves. I believe much of the decision making and responsibility belong to the patient rather than the doctor. For my part, I try to provide nonabrasive guidance.

Kevin is keeping his weight down, which I regard as a good sign.

• • •

Dangers of a Protein-Rich, Low-Carb Diet

Apart from vitamin B deficiencies, high homocysteine levels can be caused by diets rich in animal protein. As previously mentioned, homocysteine is derived from methionine. This amino acid's most likely source is meat. Dr. McCully talked about "protein intoxication" as a cause of atherosclerosis. The protein-rich, low-carb diets presently so much in favor can potentially boost your homocysteine level—and therefore your risk of heart disease.

Dr. Nancy Green, the medical director of the March of Dimes, said that the foundation is concerned about the increasing popularity of low-carb diets and the possibility that people will not consume as much folic acid as they need if they avoid fortified bread and cereals. "It's hard to know what the effect of these low-carb diets is going to be," she told *The Wall Street Journal*, "but we're very nervous about this."

I don't know of any reports that prove a connection between any protein-rich, low-carb diet and elevated homocysteine levels. All the same, I do not hesitate to tell patients with high homocysteine levels to limit red meat in general. You can cut back on starches, refined grains, and simple sugars without your diet becoming too protein-rich. I'm in favor of balance in diet and exercise.

Needless to say, people on a protein-rich, low-carb diet for any length of time need to keep an eye on their homocysteine levels.

What to Do About
High Homocysteine

Exercise and B-complex vitamins lower your homocysteine and C-reactive protein levels. For men and women aged 60 to 80 years, six months of resistance exercises reduced the homocysteine levels by more than 5 percent, in a University of Virginia study led by Dr. K. R. Vincent.

In a Massachusetts neighborhood, fruit and vegetable intake was matched with homocysteine and C-reactive protein levels for 445 Hispanic elderly people and 154 non-Hispanic white elderly people. You guessed it—those with the highest fruit and vegetable intake had the lowest homocysteine and C-reactive protein levels. At some future time, we will discover the ailments caused by a diet deficient in the vitamins, minerals, and micronutrients found in fresh fruit and vegetables. This nutritional lack is suffered most severely by children and growing young people.

Dr. David J. DeRose of the Lifestyle Center of America in Sulphur, Oklahoma, depended on diet alone, without the use of vitamin B supplements, to lower the homocysteine levels of forty men and women in a study lasting one week. Completely avoiding all animal products, caffeine, and alcohol, they reduced their levels by an average of 13 percent in that time.

Do Vitamin B Supplements Work?

If your high homocysteine level is a result of a vitamin B deficiency, can supplements of folic acid, B-6, and B-12 lower it and protect you against heart disease? Some doctors say yes, and others say it has not been proved. If the remedy was expensive or dangerous, I would give this matter a lot of thought before recommending it to a patient. But vitamin B supplements are inexpensive and safe. If you have a high homocysteine level, take folic acid, B-6, and B-12 at the recommended doses.

But do supplements work? They did for participants in a study by Dr. Daniel G. Hackam and colleagues at the Siebens-Drake/Robarts Research Institute in London, Ontario. Taking 2.5 milligrams of folic acid, 25 milligrams of B-6, and 250 micrograms of B-12 every day for a year slowed and even reversed clogging of the carotid arteries, which bring blood to the brain, reducing the risk of a stroke. Dr. Hackam suggested that for people who already have cardiovascular disease, a homocysteine level of 9 (normal for a healthy person) may need to be lowered. Once again, homocysteine resembles cholesterol in that its optimal lowest level remains unknown.

A British study in 2002 showed that a daily intake of 800 micrograms (twice the RDA) of folic acid significantly lowers the risk of heart disease, stroke, and deep-vein thrombosis. On the other hand, according to another study, taking daily doses of 2.5 milligrams (more than six times the RDA) of folic acid did not help reduce the recurrence of strokes in people who had already had one. But the lead researcher in this study, Dr. James F. Toole, director of the Stroke Research Center at Wake Forest University in Winston-Salem, North Carolina, believes in a prevention strategy against strokes of starting to take high doses of folic acid in your thirties, rather than waiting until your sixties.

Taking B Supplements

Do you get enough vitamin B? It depends on the foods you eat. (See Chapter 6, pages 61–63, for a list of foods.)

I advise patients with high homocysteine levels to cut back on meat, coffee, and alcohol. Vitamin B derived from food alone would rarely be sufficient to lower high homocysteine levels, so I recommend taking supplements. Take twice the daily minimum requirements in B-complex form for several months.

If dietary precautions and supplements are not enough to lower a patient's homocysteine level to near normal over a course of months—it normally takes at least three months—I may prescribe a higher-dose vitamin B preparation.

8. Fasting Insulin Test

FASTING INSULIN TEST

What Is It?

A blood test to measure the level of the hormone insulin

Test Results

Above 25 micro international units per milliliter (μIU/mL) of blood	High risk
15–25 μIU/mL	Borderline high risk
Below 15 μIU/mL	Normal

Cost Without Medical Insurance

About $75

Of a number of insulin tests, the fasting insulin test is the easiest to perform and the most convenient for the patient. You fast for eight hours before the test. I find that most people prefer to be tested in the morning after fasting from midnight.

The results of this test are complicated by the different scoring systems of various medical laboratories. Keep in mind that your doctor's lab may use a different but equally valid scoring system than was used for the results given above. He or she will be able to interpret the results for you.

High levels of insulin in your bloodstream cause a wide range of damage to your body's tissues, although it's not always clear whether the insulin itself causes the damage or is simply a marker of the process. Dr. Gerald Reaven, the discoverer of the metabolic syndrome (which he called "syndrome X"), believes that all its health problems can ultimately be traced back to high insulin levels. As you probably know, heart disease is the frequent end result of the metabolic syndrome.

Insulin Resistance

You are most likely to have a high insulin level because of insulin resistance, which is an inherited tendency. However, the health consequences of insulin resistance can be modified by weight loss and exercise, and for most people with insulin resistance, as long as they do not become overweight and inactive, their insulin levels will not become high. Insulin enables your cells to take in glucose from your blood to use as fuel for energy. If your cells become less sensitive (more resistant) to insulin, more insulin will be required to handle the same amounts of glucose. With increasing insulin resistance, higher levels of insulin and eventually glucose will be found in the blood.

It was once thought that a fasting glucose test would reveal insulin resistance. Now it is known, again through Dr. Reaven of Stanford University, that you can be insulin-resistant and have a normal result on a fasting glucose test. This is because your increased insulin level has compensated for your insulin resistance and kept your blood glucose at a normal level. Although the result is within a normal range, your high insulin level is insidiously damaging your body tissues.

Insulin resistance has multiple links to heart disease, mostly by way of the metabolic syndrome.

A "tight coupling" exists between insulin resistance and arterial wall damage, according to Dr. John P. Cooke of Stanford University. The cells lining the artery wall begin to behave differently in people with high insulin levels. For example, an artery's ability to widen and narrow with blood flow is lessened. Exercise decreases these negative effects, and obesity increases them, according to Dr. H. O. Steinberg and coworkers.

High Insulin Levels and Arterial Inflammation

When you eat too much, insulin stores some of the blood glucose you don't use for energy as fat. Fat cells, although outside the vascular system, can contribute to inflammation inside arteries. A number of substances active in arterial inflammation are secreted by fat cells, including C-reactive protein. While most CRP is made by the liver, fat cells can secrete dangerous quantities. The same holds true for other substances. Additionally, in a vicious circle, fat cells secrete substances that make insulin resistance worse and insulin levels higher, leading to the formation of more fat cells and the secretion of more inflammation-promoting substances. Fat cells can even decrease the levels of anti-inflammatory agents such as adiponectin, as shown by J. G. Yu and colleagues at Umea University in Sweden. Doctors agree that much has yet to be learned about the complex links between high insulin levels, insulin resistance, and arterial inflammation.

• NATALIE'S STORY •

Natalie, 31, had a family history of type 2 (adult-onset) diabetes. Twenty years ago, it would have been unusual for someone Natalie's age to develop this kind of diabetes. Today refined carbs, inactivity, and obesity have produced an epidemic of type 2 diabetes among people in their twenties and thirties, and even in their teens. Natalie was overweight, lived on soda and junk food, and never walked when she could drive. Her results from fasting glucose and two-hour glucose tolerance tests were poor. Her triglyceride level was high, but her LDL, HDL, and total cholesterol levels were nearly normal. Her mother, a diabetic survivor of two major heart attacks, asked me to talk to her.

The result of Natalie's fasting insulin test confirmed her earlier poor glucose results. Her insulin level of 32 predicted that she might not have to wait long for some serious health problems to appear. I described some of them to her in realistic detail. Knowing that she lived at home with her mother, I was not optimistic about any lifestyle changes.

But Natalie did not want what had happened to her mother to happen to her, and she did something about it. On subsequent visits, her dropping weight and increased activity were matched by dropping insulin levels and rebounding health. Natalie has succeeded in keeping at bay the development of type 2 diabetes. She is presently working on her mother to improve her lifestyle and health.

• • •

What You Can Do About a High Insulin Level

Because insulin resistance is probably the cause of your high insulin level and is also the main cause of type 2 diabetes, preventive strategies for prediabetics and type 2 diabetics will benefit you. In a study called the Diabetes Prevention Program, a 7 percent weight loss and 150 minutes a week of moderate exercise reduced diabetes by 58 percent. Most doctors regard a weight loss of 5 to 10 percent as realistic—meaning that you can achieve it without monumental effort and can keep the weight off without much stress. The immediate results are noticeable improvements in health, energy, fitness, well-being, and self-esteem, which is quite a lot for such a small effort.

9. Ferritin Test

FERRITIN TEST

What Is It?

A blood test to measure the level of the protein ferritin

Test Results

Males: 12–300 nanograms per milliliter (ng/mL) of blood	Normal
Females: 12–150 ng/mL	Normal

Cost Without Medical Insurance

About $85

Raises Ferritin Level

Alcoholic liver disease

Breast cancer

Chronic inflammation (rheumatoid arthritis, inflammatory bowel disease, bacterial infections)

Hemochromatosis

Hemolytic anemia

Hyperthyroidism

Iron deficiency anemia

Iron overload states

Iron supplements

Leukemia

Liver disease

Lymphoma

Megablastic anemia

Neuroblastomas

Other kinds of anemia

Lowers Ferritin Level

Chronic gastrointestinal bleeding

Heavy menstrual bleeding

Iron deficiency anemia

The body uses the protein ferritin as its chief way to store iron for making hemoglobin and other iron-containing proteins. Ferritin is found in high concentrations in many tissues. The blood level of ferritin has been shown to reflect the amount of iron stored in the body. Thus this test is important for detecting disorders associated with either iron overload or deficiency.

About 30 percent of the world population is iron-deficient, mostly women and children. One in ten American women and small children were found to be iron-deficient in 1997. Concern over possible iron deficiency is very often the reason why people have their ferritin levels tested. If your test result shows that you have a low ferritin level, your doctor will recommend therapy for iron deficiency. Your low level is not indicative of cardiovascular disease, but a high iron level can indicate a problem.

High Ferritin Levels and
Iron Overload

Iron overload is much less common than iron deficiency. A high ferritin level indicates that the body is storing too much iron in the tissues. Excess iron in tissues has been associated with heart disease for decades. The iron content of the body rises because the mineral is not excreted or broken down in the way that many other minerals are. A very small quantity of iron is lost in urine, sweat, and dead cells, some is consumed in tissue growth, and some is lost in menstrual bleeding. It has even been suggested that the menstrual loss of excess iron by women may be as important as the presence of estrogen in protecting them from heart attacks.

An explanation for the connection between a high ferritin level due to excess iron in your tissues and atherosclerosis was offered by a researcher from Finland, Dr. Jukka Salonen, in 1992. Unused iron courses through the body in the form of free radicals, ready to combine with tissue substances by oxidizing them. LDL particles embedded in an artery wall build plaque by becoming oxidized. In this way, excess iron can be said to enable LDL to cause harm.

High Ferritin Levels, Arterial
Inflammation, and Insulin Resistance

A high ferritin level can also be caused by inflammation rather than excess iron in tissues. Perhaps the body, on detecting inflammation, supplies extra ferritin to the blood for making new hemoglobin to replace that lost in potential bleeding from the supposed wound. Results from CRP and fibrinogen tests could confirm inflammation as the cause. Regardless of its cause, a high ferritin level puts you at cardiac risk and it is important to bring that level down.

Ferritin can be a cause as well as a marker of inflammation. One form of ferritin, known as "ferritin light chain," may promote oxidation of LDL in the artery wall through the generation of highly reactive oxygen particles, according to Dr. S. A. You and colleagues at the Cleveland Clinic. LDL oxidation in the artery wall produces oxysterols as a by-product. Ferritin levels and oxysterols were found to be linked in 669 men by Dr. T. P. Tuomainen and colleagues at the University of Kuopio, Finland.

Very recent research suggests that we don't know the whole story of ferritin levels in the blood and iron storage in the body. Using the nearly 33,000 women who provided blood samples for the Nurses' Health Study, Dr. Rui Jiang and Harvard colleagues found that higher iron stores, as reflected by elevated ferritin levels, caused increased risk of type 2 diabetes. The researchers noted that women who developed diabetes also usually had high scores from CRP and fasting insulin tests. Most diabetics die of heart disease.

In another study, high ferritin levels have been linked to glucose intolerance and insulin resistance in healthy people by Dr. Michael Haap and colleagues.

Are there links between ferritin, CRP, and cholesterol? This question was answered by Dr. A. G. Mainous III and colleagues at the Medical University of South Carolina in Charleston. Their study found that people with high ferritin and high LDL were likely to have high CRP. Further, they showed that people with high ferritin and low HDL were also likely to have high CRP. You could infer from this that arterial inflammation is induced by high ferritin plus high bad cholesterol or low good cholesterol.

Broad Normal Range

The extensive normal range for ferritin of 12 to 300 ng/mL for men and 12 to 150 for women is unusual. The lower the ferritin level in this broad range of normal values, the greater the likelihood the person is iron-deficient. The level at which ferritin becomes a cardiac risk is a matter of judgment for doctors. I do not use an absolute number, either in men or women. I become watchful when I see a level above 200 in men and above 100 in women. I become increasingly concerned as levels build.

Iron-Rich Diets

The Harvard researchers noted that the women with high ferritin levels who developed diabetes tended to have a family history of diabetes, exercised less, drank more alcohol, and had a higher intake of total calories. They also ate more trans fats, red meat, processed meats, and heme iron (iron in its natural form in food, as distinct from the synthetic non-heme form of supplements). They ingested less cereal fiber and magnesium.

Iron as a mineral is not easily absorbed by humans from un-enriched cereals. That iron can be nutritionally absorbed from soybeans in the form of ferritin was demonstrated by Laura E. Murray-Kolb and colleagues at Penn State, Cornell, and the Children's Hospital Oakland Research Institute in California. In the study eighteen women, most with a slight iron deficiency, ate soup and muffins made from soybeans. This made their blood levels of ferritin rise significantly. This, of course, would be beneficial if you had an iron deficiency, and disastrous if you already had a high ferritin level.

The following foods are rich in iron: eggs, fish, liver, red meat, poultry, green leafy vegetables, soy, whole grains, and enriched breads and cereals. But iron occurs to some extent in such a wide array of foods, it is nearly impossible to avoid. If you have a high ferritin level, don't eat liver, red meat, soy products, and iron-enriched foods.

• DAVID'S STORY •

During his forties, David let his body go, ignoring an expanding waistline and increasing body weight. As a tax lawyer, he put in long hours of sedentary work. His way of relaxing at the end of the day was to sink into an armchair with a glass of wine and listen to music. After his wife left, the time he spent with music and wine increased.

In his late fifties, he remarried. Then, at 61, he developed a chest pain that steadily grew worse. His doctor diagnosed it as unstable angina—the dangerous kind—and referred him to me.

David's lipid panel results were all normal, but his CRP level was a little elevated. His ferritin level was high. I told him that his chances of avoiding a heart attack did not look good as long as his angina remained unstable—that is, as it worsened.

In this country, most cases of unstable angina are dealt with through intervention. David received cardiac catheterization. He was found to have moderate disease in two coronary arteries. In his third coronary artery, he had 80 percent blockage and what appeared to be unstable plaque. He underwent balloon angioplasty, and a stent was put in place in the artery. After the procedure, he took vitamins daily and became more active. As his activity increased and his weight dropped, his anginal pain continued to diminish until it disappeared.

His ferritin level slowly decreased as he regained his health, but it had served him well by serving as a warning light when it mattered most.

• • •

10. Lipoprotein(a) Test

LIPOPROTEIN(A) TEST

What Is It?

A blood test to measure the level of lipoprotein(a)

Test Results

Above 19 milligrams per deciliter (mg/dL) of blood	High risk
14–19 mg/dL	Borderline high risk
Below 14 mg/dL	Normal

Cost Without Medical Insurance

About $75

Lipoprotein(a), pronounced "lipoprotein little a" or "L-P little a," is made by the liver. As a lipoprotein, it is a combination of a lipid and a protein, in this case an LDL cholesterol particle attached to a plasminogen-like molecule. Plasminogen is the precursor of the enzyme plasmin, which breaks down and digests blood clots. Lp(a) is about 40 percent LDL cholesterol by weight.

Lp(a) contributes to atherosclerosis in four ways: (1) it slows down the breakup of blood clots; (2) it promotes the formation of clots; (3) it helps macrophages to turn into foam cells in the artery wall; and (4) it promotes the proliferation of smooth muscle cells in the artery wall, enlarging plaque. Lp(a) probably also transports cholesterol to the plaque site. It's not known exactly why we have Lp(a) in our bodies in the first place. It probably helps by responding to tissue injury, preventing infectious agents from invading cells and promoting wound healing.

Numerous studies have confirmed the links between high Lp(a) levels and atherosclerosis, heart attacks, and strokes. The association between Lp(a) and atherosclerosis at least partly involves high LDL levels. About 37 percent of Americans at high risk for developing coronary artery disease have an elevated Lp(a) level, while only 14 percent of low-risk people have one. The higher the Lp(a) level, the more severe the coronary artery disease. Although Lp(a) is an independent cardiac risk factor, someone who has an elevated Lp(a) level also often has an elevated homocysteine level.

Threat of Small Apo(a) Particle

The most important role of Lp(a) in heart disease is its ability to slow down the breakup of blood clots. The protein part of this lipoprotein is responsible. Called "apolipoprotein(a)" or "apo(a)," it very closely resembles plasminogen, the precursor of the enzyme plasmin, which breaks down the fibrin in blood clots. Apo(a) binds with fibrin in the clot in the place of plasminogen, lengthening the clot's existence. In addition, the presence of this plasminogen-like substance probably causes lesser amounts of genuine plasminogen to be secreted to clear a clot.

Your Lp(a) level and the size of the apo(a) particle are inherited. Apo(a) substantially varies in size among people. Small apo(a) particles bind with clot fibrin more readily than large apo(a) particles. If you have inherited small apo(a), as well as a high Lp(a) level, you have a much higher cardiac risk. Your doctor can go over this with you when the lab test result comes in.

What Doctors Have Learned About Lp(a)

In the Physicians' Health Study, men with the highest levels of Lp(a) and LDL were twelve times as likely to develop angina as men with the lowest levels, according to Dr. N. Rifai and colleagues at the Harvard Medical School. They found Lp(a) to be an excellent predictor of angina in healthy men, particularly when combined with a high LDL level.

Cardiovascular Health Study researchers led by Dr. Abraham A. Ariyo found Lp(a) to be a predictor of heart disease in elderly men but not women. They measured the Lp(a) level in blood samples from 2,375 women and 1,597 men aged 65 or older. Of the men, those with the highest Lp(a) levels had three times the risk of stroke, almost three times the risk of death from cardiovascular disease, and nearly twice the risk of death from all causes, compared to those with the lowest Lp(a) levels. Although no relationship was found for elderly women in this study, this has not been the case in other studies.

In Japan, 208 people aged 80, suffering from a variety of illnesses, were examined to see how their Lp(a) levels corresponded to their diseases. A high Lp(a) level strongly correlated with lipid-rich, unstable plaque in the carotid arteries. The Tokyo Medical University Hospital researchers found that an inherited elevated Lp(a) level could promote atherosclerosis throughout a person's life and become an independent cardiovascular risk factor later in life.

Who Is Likely to Have a High Lp(a) Level

The amount of Lp(a) in your blood is about 90 percent genetically determined. Its level is not affected by the foods you eat or how much you exercise. People with familial hypercholesterolemia are particularly likely to have a high Lp(a) blood level.

Mothers with children who have high Lp(a) levels are twice as likely to have a heart attack as other mothers. In Spain, 6-year-old children whose grandparents had died of stroke or coronary artery disease had significantly higher levels of Lp(a).

Lp(a) varies with race, according to Dr. H. D. Wu and colleagues at Columbia University in New York City. African Americans have the highest levels, Hispanics intermediate levels, and Caucasians the lowest levels. The physicians noted that although the Lp(a) level has been shown to be a reliable predictor of heart disease in Caucasians, much less is known about its performance as a predictor in non-Caucasians.

What Can You Do About It?

Neomycin and nicotinic acid are the only cholesterol-lowering drugs that also lower Lp(a) levels. Estrogen supplements are known to lower Lp(a) levels.

Many doctors believe that the best way to lower your Lp(a) level may be to lower your LDL level. Some doctors recommend small doses of aspirin. Lowering high homocysteine levels with B-complex vitamins can also have a beneficial effect on Lp(a) levels. Lowering high blood pressure may help too.

• ISABEL'S STORY •

On turning 50, Isabel declared victory on having gone through menopause without resorting to hormone replacement therapy. But on each of her last three annual checkups, her LDL level had steadily climbed, though still remaining within the normal range. Her doctor referred her to me.

I ran another series of tests. Isabel's LDL had climbed again—it was now a high normal. Her homocysteine level was high, and at 23 mg/dL, so was her Lp(a). Neither level had been tested before. Her HDL and total cholesterol levels were normal, though like her LDL, just barely.

We know that Lp(a) empowers LDL to attack arterial walls and build plaque. Homocysteine plays a role in this also. In the absence of estrogen's protection, the combination of all three could lead to the development of plaque in coronary and other arteries. After Isabel received therapy, the levels of all three dropped.

• • •

Natural Remedy to Lower Lp(a)

It has been theorized that both Lp(a) and cholesterol are manufactured by the liver to repair tiny fissures in the walls of aging blood vessels. Both of these lipoproteins have the ability to patch such fissures. One way to persuade the liver not to make so much Lp(a) and cholesterol, the theory claims, is to provide the body with plenty of collagen, which can also patch the fissures. A cocktail of vitamin C, L-lysine, and L-proline provides the body with the makings of large amounts of collagen, which should help keep artery walls clear of Lp(a) and cholesterol and reduce the blood levels of both.

Primates, including humans, are some of the few animals, apart from guinea pigs and fruit-eating bats, that don't manufacture vitamin C inside their own bodies. They are also the only animals with Lp(a) in their blood. Dr. Linus Pauling and Dr. Mathias Rath regarded Lp(a) as a fallback mechanism for those animals when they could not get enough vitamin C in their food. They found that guinea pigs deprived of vitamin C accumulated Lp(a) in plaque in damaged arteries. When the guinea pigs were given abundant vitamin C, they didn't develop plaque in damaged arteries.

They also found that the amino acid lysine—another ingredient of the cocktail—somehow inactivated Lp(a) without lowering its blood level.

It is difficult to estimate the dose of vitamin C needed by humans.

11. Calcium Heart Scan

CALCIUM HEART SCAN

What Is It?

A CT scan of the heart to detect deposits of the mineral calcium

Test Results

Above 400	You need an exercise stress test to check if plaque in your coronary arteries is impeding blood flow to your heart muscle
Above 300	Major plaque buildup
100 to 300	Moderate plaque buildup
0	No detectable plaque

Cost Without Medical Insurance

$250–$600

I n May 2003, the former New York Knicks basketball star Dave DeBusschere was walking to lunch in downtown Manhattan. Although 62 years old, the 6-foot-6 ex-athlete was still fit. He was not much above his playing weight and had no known health problems or symptoms. Without warning, he fell to the sidewalk and died of a heart attack.

More than 260,000 Americans die each year from heart attacks. Nearly half of them, like Dave DeBusschere, have no symptoms of coronary artery disease and die without advance warning. Their first symptom kills them.

You might need to keep that in mind when you consider the cost of calcium heart screening. The previously discussed tests, performed on a blood sample, are less expensive and thus less likely to be challenged by your medical insurance company. A screening calcium heart scan, at a cost of $250 to $600, is unlikely to be paid for by your medical insurance provider. Your insurance company may demand a preliminary diagnosis of cardiac symptoms from your doctor before you have a scan.

You don't need a doctor's referral to have a heart scan. But if you walk into an imaging center on your own, without a referral, you further reduce your chances of reimbursement by your health insurance.

At the Imaging Center

You are most likely to have your heart screened at a commercial imaging center. As well as heart scans, most centers do whole-body scans for cancer. CT scans are computer-enhanced x-ray images revealing structures that would not show up on an ordinary x-ray.

You can have your heart scanned in two ways: by electron-beam CT or by helical CT. In helical CT, the most available kind, the x-ray camera spins around your body and takes shots from all angles. However, because more medical data exist for electron-beam CT, it's preferable to have this kind of screening.

For an electron-beam scan, you lie on your back on a movable table. A technician attaches electrodes to your chest. Then the remote-controlled table slides feetfirst into the scanner, leaving your head outside. For about a minute, you lie absolutely still and listen to a series of clicks in the machine. Then the table slides out again, this time headfirst. The scan is finished, and the technician removes the electrodes from your chest. There's no image for you to see. Your results have to be analyzed by an expert, so don't expect to hear anything for almost a week.

Finding an Imaging Center

Many doctors believe that CT medical imaging is only in its infancy. Most cities have commercial imaging enters independent of the local hospitals, and new ones are opening all the time. Your doctor can recommend one or you can probably find several in any phone book. Major medical centers are now competing by offering more sophisticated CT scanners than those in small commercial imaging centers. Some of the new CT scanners have as many as sixty-four detectors compared to the four or fewer detectors of older scanners. A question worth asking is whether the center has one of the new scanners made by Siemens, Toshiba, General Electric, and Philips. Safety? That very much depends on precautions taken by the staff. If the center appears to be very well run and highly organized, it's reasonable to assume that the staff is meticulous about safety precautions.

Why Calcium?

Why scan for calcium? The mineral calcium is deposited—along with cholesterol, other lipids, and cell detritus—in plaque that forms in artery walls. The amount and density of calcium in your heart scan indicate how much plaque you have in your coronary arteries, which lie on the surface of your heart. There is no "good" arterial calcium. The only reason for any to show in a scan is that it is embedded in plaque. In a heart scan, if you have calcium, you have plaque. It's as simple as that.

The amount of calcium in your heart scan is known as your calcium score. The higher your score, the greater the *risk* of a coronary blockage that can lead to a heart attack.

Heart Scans as Predictors

Heart scans were given to 5,000 men and women with no cardiac symptoms by Dr. George T. Kondos, associate chief of cardiology at the University of Illinois at Chicago. The men with the highest calcium scores were almost 2.5 times as likely to have a heart attack as all the men with moderate and low scores. The highest-scoring men were more than ten times as likely to need angioplasty or by-pass surgery. Dr. Kondos told *The New York Times* that calcium heart scanning helps him decide how aggressively to treat "an intermediate group—men over 45 with one or two risk factors, the same for women over 50—whose ten-year risk of a heart attack is between 10 and 15 percent." At least a third of American adults belong to this group that is intermediate between low and high cardiac risk groups.

Researchers at Northwestern, UCLA, and the University of

Southern California also found heart scans valuable is assessing treatment for intermediate-risk people. They gave heart scans to 1,312 Californians over 45—most were in their sixties. They followed up on their health for an average of seven years, during which time 84 either had a heart attack or died from heart-related causes. They found calcium heart scans to be an excellent predictor of cardiac events. When people have an intermediate cardiac risk, their doctors can easily assume that they don't need aggressive therapy, such as a strict diet or statins. A heart scan can either contradict or support a decision to do nothing—a decision that can prove fatal.

Like a lot of medical research, however, this California study (published in *The Journal of the American Medical Association*, or *JAMA*) did not deliver a simple answer to a simple question. The wrinkle here was that having a perfect calcium score did not mean that participants were free of cardiac risk. For example, 7 of 75 people with a calcium score of 0 but an otherwise high risk of heart attack went on to have one. So did 7 of 195 people with a 0 calcium score and an intermediate risk. One lesson in this is that you can't place all your reliance on any single test. In my practice, when possible I always back up the result of one test with that of at least one other. But these participants, of course, did have other tests, which was why the researchers knew that they had high cardiac risks in spite of their 0 calcium scores. For me, the real lesson here is that the risk factor that you *don't* have does not protect you from the risk factors that you *do* have.

12. A New Look
at the Old Tests

Cholesterol: How Low
Should You Go?

The fact that many people with normal cholesterol levels have heart attacks indicates that the so-called normal level is too high, according to a number of cardiologists. They believe that the normal total cholesterol level ceiling should have been lowered from 240 to 160, instead of 200. One good reason for not having done so, they acknowledge, is that it would have caused a sizable portion of the American population to become discouraged.

The results of the Minnesota Heart Survey show that the United States still has a long way to go in cholesterol awareness and treatment. This survey of more than 5,000 people in Minneapolis and St. Paul is taken every five years. For the period

2000–2002, the survey found the following for adults with high cholesterol aged 25 to 74:

	Women	Men
Unaware of their high cholesterol:	32%	32%
Aware, but high cholesterol untreated:	35%	24%
High cholesterol being treated:	28%	41%
Cholesterol treatment not working:	5%	3%

We are born with a total cholesterol level of less than 100. If, throughout our whole lives, we never ate hamburgers, french fries, mayonnaise, and similar foods, our cholesterol levels might remain at around this level. This would minimize the risk of cardiovascular disease over our lifetimes. We don't know the level for total cholesterol below which it would be unhealthy to go. The substance cholesterol is used in building cells and other body processes—we need it to keep alive. Although we don't know the lower level of how much cholesterol we need—that is, the lowest limit for healthy total cholesterol—we know with certainty that the desirable upper level is below 160.

I have mentioned previously that our increasing ability to get LDL down to very low levels may be associated with an increase in cognitive problems. I have even seen a couple of cases of dementia in people in their late forties. It's not known if statins or other LDL-reducing drugs are responsible for the cognitive problems or if the lowered cholesterol level itself is at fault.

It may be relevant that the brain is made up mostly of cholesterol. Peripheral nerves are "insulated" with cholesterol in the way that electrical wires are with plastic. These facts should not cause us to jump to conclusions, but they cannot be ignored.

Home Testing of Cholesterol

Home cholesterol tests are becoming widely available, as people worry about the consequences of high-fat, no-carb diets. Most of the home tests require you to prick your finger with a lancet and apply the drop of blood to a test strip. A survey by *The Wall Street Journal* of five kits available in early 2004 found that home results differed significantly from commercial lab results from the same sample. The survey faulted all five kits for this lack of reliability.

Expect your cholesterol level to vary with seasonal temperatures. In Massachusetts, where winter is really winter, people's cholesterol levels are apt to rise by 4 to 6 in the coldest months. Density changes in the blood plasma may be responsible, according to Dr. Ira S. Ockene of the University of Massachusetts Medical Center.

Cholesterol Blood Levels and Heart Disease Risk

Total Cholesterol Level

240 or more	High risk
200–239	Borderline high risk
Below 200	Desirable

LDL Cholesterol Level

190 or more	Very high risk
160–189	High risk
130–159	Borderline high risk
100–129	Near optimal
Below 100	Optimal

HDL Cholesterol Level

Below 40	Risk factor for heart disease
60 or more	Protects against heart disease

SOURCE: National Cholesterol Education Program.

LDL Level and Risk Factors

The guidelines issued by the federal government's National Cholesterol Education Program concentrate on lowering your LDL cholesterol level instead of your total cholesterol level. The third edition of the guidelines stresses two main prevention strategies:

1. If you are healthy, you can prevent heart disease by reducing your intake of saturated fats and cholesterol, increasing your physical activity, and controlling your weight.
2. If you already have coronary artery disease, you can prevent further cardiac events by getting your LDL level below 100.

The guidelines were written to help doctors, not to tell them what to do. Apparently some doctors follow the guidelines more closely than others. People complain that their doctors don't seem to follow the guidelines and don't take time to explain what goals the patients should aim for. No doubt some doctors feel that the issues are too complex for a simple explanation—or that they did indeed explain and their patients did not understand. To ensure that you have the essential information on who should reduce LDL and by how much, I have given some of the basics here. You can find this information in greater detail at the National Cholesterol Education Program's Web site at www.nhlbi .nih.gov/guidelines/cholesterol/atp_iii.htm.

The focus is on LDL levels because they are among the best indicators we have of heart health. The guidelines divide people with elevated LDL into three categories and suggest the appropriate therapy for each category. The percentage risk of heart disease over ten years is calculated from the Framingham study point scores. You can estimate yours from the tables that follow the category descriptions (see pages 107–109).

Category 1

The people who belong here have coronary artery disease already or a greater than 20 percent risk of it in ten years. They make up the highest risk group. Their LDL goal is a level of less than 100. Lifestyle changes can help. At LDL levels of 100 to 129, drug therapy is optional. At 130 or above, it is suggested.

Category 2

The people in this category have two or more cardiac risk factors or a 20 percent or less risk of heart disease in ten years. Their LDL goal is below 130. Diet and exercise can help.

Those with a 10 to 20 percent risk in ten years should consider drug therapy at an LDL level of 130 or more.

Those with a less then 10 percent risk in ten years should consider drug therapy at 160 or more.

Category 3

The people here have one or no cardiac risk factors but have an LDL level of 160 or more. They need to get their levels below 160. Lifestyle changes alone may be sufficient to achieve this. At levels 160 to 189, drug therapy is optional. At 190 or above, it is suggested.

New Recommendations

Changes to these recommendations were suggested in a July 2004 National Cholesterol Education Program report, with Dr. Scott M. Grundy as its lead author.

- An LDL level of below 70 is recommended for people with very high risk.
- When people with high risk have high triglyceride or low HDL levels, they should consider combining a fibrate or niacin with their LDL-lowering drug.
- The LDL goal of 130 for category 2 people should be lowered to 100.
- When you start taking an LDL-lowering drug, its dosage should be powerful enough to lower your LDL level by 30 to 40 percent.

The following tables depict men's risk of heart disease in ten-year periods, using Framingham point scores. The total number of points will give you a risk percentage.

Age	20–34	35–39	40–44	45–49	50–54	55–59	60–64	65–69	70–74	75–79
Points	−9	−4	0	3	6	8	10	11	12	13

Total Cholesterol	Age 20–39	Age 40–49	Age 50–59	Age 60–69	Age 70–79
159 or less	0	0	0	0	0
160–199	4	3	2	1	0
200–239	7	5	3	1	0
240–279	9	6	4	2	1
280 or more	11	8	5	3	1

	Age 20–39	Age 40–49	Age 50–59	Age 60–69	Age 70–79
Nonsmoker	0	0	0	0	0
Smoker	8	5	3	1	1

HDL	60 or more	50–59	40–49	39 or less
Points	−1	0	1	2

Systolic Blood Pressure	Untreated	Treated
119 or less	0	0
120–129	0	1
130–139	1	2
140–159	1	2
160 or more	2	3

Total Points	% Risk in 10 Years	Total Points	% Risk in 10 Years
0	1	9	5
1	1	10	6
2	1	11	8
3	1	12	10
4	1	13	12
5	2	14	16
6	2	15	20
7	3	16	25
8	4	17 or more	30 or more

The following tables depict women's risk of heart disease in ten-year periods, using Framingham point scores. The total number of points will give you a risk percentage.

Age	20–34	35–39	40–44	45–49	50–54	55–59	60–64	65–69	70–74	75–79
Points	−7	−3	0	3	6	8	10	12	14	16

Total Cholesterol	Age 20–39	Age 40–49	Age 50–59	Age 60–69	Age 70–79
159 or less	0	0	0	0	0
160–199	4	3	2	1	1
200–239	8	6	4	2	1
240–279	11	8	5	3	2
280 or more	13	10	7	4	2
Nonsmoker	0	0	0	0	0
Smoker	9	7	4	2	1

HDL	60 or more	50–59	40–49	39 or less
Points	−1	0	1	2

Systolic Blood Pressure	Untreated	Treated
119 or less	0	0
120–129	1	3
130–139	2	4
140–159	3	5
160 or more	4	6

Total Points	% Risk in 10 Years	Total Points	% Risk in 10 Years
9	1	18	6
10	1	19	8
11	1	20	11
12	1	21	14
13	2	22	17
14	2	23	22
15	3	24	27
16	4	25 or more	30 or more
17	5		

Information Sources

You can get free information on cholesterol and other aspects of cardiovascular health from the following national organizations.

American Heart Association
7272 Greenville Avenue
Dallas, TX 75231
800-242-8721
www.americanheart.org

Centers for Disease Control and Prevention
Division of Nutrition and Physical Activity and Health Promotion
7440 Buford Highway, NE-MS/K-24
Atlanta, GA 30341-3717
770-488-5820
www.cdc.gov/nccdphp/dnpa

National Cholesterol Education Program
National Heart, Lung and Blood Institute Health Information Center
P.O. Box 30105
Bethesda, MD 20824-0105
www.nhlbi.nih.gov/chd

National Coalition for Women with Heart Disease
www.womenheart.org

Lifestyle Changes vs. Drug Therapy

For each of the three categories, lifestyle changes can help to lower LDL levels. Even when lifestyle changes are not sufficient in themselves to achieve the desired LDL level, they help lower its level and can reduce the drug dosage necessary.

My advice is to try hard at making lifestyle changes before you resort to the option of drug therapy. It's never a wise choice to take a drug simply because you won't make the effort required for a more healthy life. On the other hand, don't put off needed drug therapy with good intentions that you probably will never fulfill. You can always start medication and then, as your lifestyle changes begin to make their benefits felt, you can wean yourself off the drugs.

How low should your LDL level go? In a study sponsored by a drug company, plaque growth in heart patients' arteries progressed slowly at an LDL level of about 110, but stopped at about 80. We need to wait for the results of other studies to confirm this. In the meantime, don't waste any time in getting your LDL down to 80 or so.

Can Good Cholesterol Make Up for Bad?

The one blood lipid level that you are not asked to lower is your HDL. For once, higher is better. The only problem is that your HDL can be as reluctant to climb as your LDL to descend. In fact, bringing down your LDL can also lower your HDL. This happens when you reduce fat in your food and replace it with carbohydrates without also reducing the number of calories you take in. It can cause your HDL level to fall by as much as 20 percent.

Our understanding of high-density lipoprotein (HDL), or "good," cholesterol began with the Framingham Heart Study. In this study, the health of thousands of people in the Massachusetts town of Framingham was followed to see who developed cardiovascular disease. For people in this study with the same

LDL, those with higher HDL had less heart trouble than those with lower HDL.

LDL and HDL particles ferry cholesterol, but in different directions. LDL transports cholesterol to arteries, where it can become embedded in the artery walls in the form of plaque. HDL carries cholesterol to the liver, which helps excrete it from the body. In addition, HDL transports antioxidants to inflammation sites to combat LDL oxidation and plaque growth.

If your HDL was high enough, could it possibly compensate for high LDL? Could one HDL particle cancel out the effects of one LDL particle?

This was what Bob thought. A 49-year-old high school mathematics teacher in Raleigh, North Carolina, he had a high HDL level of 68. This caused him to ignore his high LDL level of 178. He came to see me for the first time after he had suffered a mild heart attack. Thinking in video game terms, he was indignant that his good cholesterol hadn't "zapped" his bad. While HDL sometimes does not function properly for unknown reasons, I said this need not necessarily be what happened in his case. From what we can see in general, I said, resorting to video game concepts myself, in a fight between the two, LDL is the stronger and will win most of the time.

"I really don't feel that treatment for high LDL should be withheld just because the HDL level is high," Dr. Daniel Rader of the University of Pennsylvania School of Medicine told *The New York Times*. He said that in judging what a patient needs, he looks at LDL and other risk factors without taking HDL into consideration. Only when the LDL and other risk factors are borderline does he allow HDL to influence his decision.

Dr. Bryan Brewer of the National Heart, Lung, and Blood Institute said, "If you have a high LDL level you should be concerned about it, independently of your HDL. You are still at risk."

Things That Lower HDL Level

Anabolic steroids
Beta blockers
High carbohydrate intake
  (more than 60 percent of calories)
High triglyceride level
Overweight
Physical inactivity
Progestational drugs
Smoking
Type 2 diabetes

Artificial HDL as Artery Drano

The technology of natural HDL infusions to decrease the volume of plaque has been in existence for two decades. HDL, however, as a natural substance, is not patentable and therefore drug companies had no incentive to develop HDL infusions for clinical use. Recently, an artificial HDL, originating from a genetic variant, has made patenting possible.

Forty-seven American heart patients were randomly assigned to be infused with either an artificial HDL or a saline solution as a control. After infusions once a week for five weeks, those who got the artificial HDL had a 4.2 percent decrease in volume of plaque in their coronary arteries. Those who got the saline had no change or a slight increase in their plaque volume.

A study with only forty-seven participants would not normally make much of an impression. But this one was led by a prominent researcher, Dr. Steven E. Nissen of the Cleveland Clinic, and its results were startling. This HDL drug had achieved in five weeks what it could take years for the bestselling LDL-lowering statin drugs to do. Besides, HDL therapy is seen as an approach to high cholesterol that has remained unexploited. The artificial HDL has been described as the medical equivalent of the plumbing cleaner Drano. It binds to cholesterol in artery wall plaque, wrenches it from the plaque, and carries it to the liver for disposal. After LDL removal, the plaque shrinks in size and stabilizes.

Because plaque takes so much time to build up, many researchers were surprised that it could be reduced in so little time. This artificial HDL infusion was ten times more powerful than the strongest statin, and statins are regarded as among the most powerful drugs for atherosclerosis.

Presently available drugs do not reliably or efficiently raise HDL levels. Fibrates and nicotinic acid (niacin) are the drugs used most often, usually by people with coronary artery disease or a high risk for it. Lowering LDL is much more likely to be seen by your doctor as a better preventive measure than raising HDL.

This artificial HDL had its origin in a remote village in northern Italy. Almost thirty years ago, two researchers discovered that although people in the village lived into their eighties and nineties and few died of cardiovascular disease, some had very low HDL levels—as low as 7 in one man. It turned out that a genetic mutation was responsible. People with the mutation actually had plenty of HDL, but it became broken down quickly after use. The mutation involved a protein called "apolipoprotein A-I," which is an HDL ingredient essential to removing LDL. An artificial form of this protein, called "ApoA-I Milano," was synthesized, and this was used in the plaque-shrinking infusions of the study.

Before it was tested in humans, ApoA-I Milano was studied in rabbits and mice by Dr. Prediman K. Shah of Cedars Sinai Medical Center in Los Angeles. It lowered the lipid content of plaque by almost one-half and also reduced inflammation of the artery wall. Its effect in mice could be seen in as little as two days.

In humans, statins are credited with reducing the risk of heart disease by about one-third. Using a statin with ApoA-I Milano might cut the risk in half. The new HDL drug is presently undergoing more widespread testing and may soon be available in Europe.

Your Triglyceride Level Seen Now as a Major Player

Triglycerides are the molecule type in which most fat exists in both your body and the food you eat. A high triglyceride blood level influences whether many people develop heart disease, especially women. "Triglycerides have a huge influence on whether women get heart disease," Dr. Thomas D. Dayspring of the University of Medicine and Dentistry of New Jersey told *Remedy* magazine. "Women who develop coronary events are more likely to have an elevation of triglycerides. We could identify a lot more women at risk if we focused on triglycerides." In causing coronary artery disease, triglycerides are linked to insulin resistance, the cause of type 2 diabetes. Your triglyceride test is separate from your cholesterol tests but is included with them in blood lipid screenings. Because your triglyceride level quickly responds to what you eat, be sure to fast for eight to twelve hours before giving a blood sample for your test.

Triglyceride Levels

500 or more	Very high
200–499	High
150–199	Borderline high
Below 150	Normal

High blood triglyceride levels are now seen as an independent risk factor for coronary artery disease. Like cholesterol, triglycerides are lipoproteins—a combination of lipid and protein. For years, triglycerides were regarded as not of much consequence, even when levels were high. Now, not only are they seen as harmful in excess, but other particles with a high triglyceride content are seen as contributors to atherosclerosis as well. Among these are remnant lipoproteins, which are partially degraded very low density lipoprotein cholesterol. Your VLDL level is regarded as a good measure of the amount of atherosclerosis-promoting remnant lipoproteins in your body.

Reaching a desirable LDL level is the primary treatment goal for everyone with an elevated triglyceride level. If your triglyceride level is borderline high (150–199), weight loss and increased physical activity are the recommended therapy. "Of all the lipids, triglycerides are most responsive to lifestyle changes, such as eating a better diet, shedding a few pounds, or putting a little exercise in your life," Dr. Dayspring said. "You may not need drugs, though you do have to be aggressive about lifestyle changes."

You need to lower a very high triglyceride level (500 or more) in order to prevent acute pancreatitis. Therapy for this requires a very low fat diet (15 percent or less calories from fats), weight loss, increased physical activity, and usually a fibrate or nicotinic acid. Excess carbohydrates in your food can also raise your triglyceride level. Only after the very high triglyceride level has been brought down at least somewhat can LDL-lowering therapy be relied upon.

Things That Increase Triglyceride Level

Beta-adrenergic blocking
agents in high doses

Chronic renal failure

Corticosteroids

Estrogen

Excess alcohol intake

High carbohydrate diet
(more than 60 percent
of calories)

Nephrotic syndrome

Overweight

Physical inactivity

Retinoids

Smoking

Some genetic lipid
disorders

Type 2 diabetes

Things That Decrease Triglyceride Level

Weight loss

Very low fat diet

Increased physical activity

Fibrates

Nicotinic acid

Statins

The Threat of Diabetes

High blood sugar associated with diabetes modifies protein macromolecules that then augment inflammatory agents in artery cell walls. Diabetes also promotes the production of oxidants that enable LDL to cause inflammatory damage. For these and other reasons, type 2 diabetes is now recognized as an independent risk factor for heart disease. The significance of such recognition lies mostly in how important it is seen from a cardiac point of view to prevent or treat the illness.

High triglycerides and low HDL are typical of people with insulin resistance, the cause of type 2 diabetes. Even so, according to the guidelines, the main target of therapy is lowering LDL.

LDL below 100: Most people with type 2 diabetes need to aim for this goal.

LDL 100 to 129: Several options exist—increasing the intensity of LDL-lowering therapy; adding a fibrate or nicotinic acid; or intensifying control of other risk factors, among them hyperglycemia.

LDL 130 or more: Most diabetics need to combine lifestyle changes with LDL-lowering drugs to achieve the goal of an LDL below 100.

LDL 200 or more: In addition to other therapy, a special effort should be made to lower the non-HDL cholesterol level.

Lifestyle Change or Drug Therapy?

One of the experts who wrote the guidelines for lowering cholesterol, Dr. Scott Grundy of the University of Texas Southwestern Medical Center, said that the committee had long discussions about trying a diet before drug therapy.

"We used to say try a diet first, but we realized that wasn't working," Dr. Grundy told *The New York Times.* "Now we say if you are at high risk, you're supposed to start drugs simultaneously with diet. For the others we used to say six months of diet. Now we say three months; we give them a chance."

It needs to be emphasized that we don't know the consequences of taking cholesterol-lowering statin drugs over an extended time. Statins have been hailed as the new aspirin, and you soon may be able to purchase them without a doctor's prescription. But once you take them to lower your LDL, you have to continue taking them to keep your LDL down. Some people start taking statins in their thirties, and make no mistake about it, doctors have no idea what the consequences for them will be if they continue taking statins into their seventies and eighties, or even before then. All drugs have side effects. Some may have few or mild short-term side effects, but more serious long-term effects. With statins, no one knows.

If you lower your LDL through weight loss, by not regaining that weight you can keep your LDL down. This is a healthier and saner way to fight cholesterol than to take drugs. That said, as a doctor who treats patients of varying commitment and willpower, I have to be practical. Like all doctors with years of clinical experience, I know that many patients sincerely commit themselves in a doctor's office to a stricter diet and more exercise than they will be able to adhere to over the following weeks and months. They mean it when they say it. However, we all have good reasons for not keeping our promises. So doctors can't allow themselves to be deceived by their patients' unrealistic good intentions.

In prescribing a cholesterol-lowering drug, I always ask for a modest commitment to weight loss through diet and exercise. If you are overweight, you have to lose only 5 to 10 percent of your body weight and take moderate exercise, such as a brisk walk for thirty minutes, at least five days a week.

Physical inactivity is a major risk factor for heart disease, interacting with other risk factors in the metabolic syndrome and impairing cardiovascular fitness and coronary blood flow. Regular moderate exercise, on the other hand, lowers LDL and VLDL and raises HDL. It also reduces blood pressure and insulin resistance.

Weight loss and activity are often sufficient in themselves to lower your LDL. When they are not, you may need a statin.

I have a hidden agenda in insisting on diet and exercise for people who take statins. While I know that diet and exercise enable statins to work better in your body, my primary reason is that more than half the people who start taking statins are no longer taking them six months later. People stop taking statins for a number of reasons: atherosclerosis is an invisible and insidious disease and they don't see any improvement; statins don't give you a lift; and the medication is expensive. Relying on statistics, I have to believe that half of my patients will not be taking their medication regularly in six months. At least they will still have the benefits of diet and exercise.

LDL-Lowering Drugs

Besides statins, three major drug types lower LDL and raise HDL: bile acid sequestrants, nicotinic acid, and fibrates. Nicotinic acid and bile acid sequestrants sometimes raise triglyceride levels. Statins slow down the liver's manufacture of cholesterol and speed up its ability to remove LDL from the blood. Bile acid sequestrants bind with cholesterol-containing bile acids in the intestine, which are then excreted in the stool. Nicotinic acid or niacin is a B vitamin. The fibrates consist of clofibrate, fenofibrate, and gemfibrozil. Of the four drug groups, statins have the fewest side effects and have delivered the best results in lowering LDL in clinical trials. This makes them the drug of choice in lowering LDL levels. They have sales of more than $13 billion in the United States. Britain, where 1.5 million people use statins, has authorized sales of at least one statin without a prescription. A Federal Drug Administration panel has denied the sale of lovastatin as an over-the-counter drug in the United States.

Two best-selling statin brands went head-to-head in publishing competing studies in November 2003. I don't intend to discuss the relative merits of the brands or even mention their names. One big difference between them was in how much they lowered LDL levels and reduced the progress of atherosclerosis.

One statin lowered LDL levels to an average of 110 and reduced disease progress to 2.7 percent over eighteen months. The other statin reduced LDL to 79, and disease progress to 0.4 percent. But the real discovery involved a subgroup in which the LDL was lowered to more or less the same level, and yet one statin outperformed the other in reducing the progress of atherosclerosis—in fact, halting it. This suggested that something other than LDL was at work. The only difference that researchers could find to account for this was that the statin that halted disease progress reduced the C-reactive protein level by 36 percent, while the other statin reduced it by only 5 percent. The anti-inflammatory effect of one statin showed what an important role C-reactive protein plays in the progress of atherosclerosis.

How Safe Are Statins?

Some of the more than 15 million Americans taking statins complain of side effects ranging from muscle pain, memory problems, weakness, fatigue, tingling or burning hands and feet, and erectile dysfunction. Muscle pain, especially in the legs, is the most frequent complaint. If this happens, you can lower the dose or try another kind of statin.

To alleviate muscle discomfort, you can also try a coenzyme Q10 supplement. The statin may be depleting this substance in your liver. Too much coenzyme Q10, however, may render your statin ineffective. A better strategy may be to take the statin in a dose low enough to be effective yet cause no muscle discomfort.

Dr. Lisa Sanders wrote in *The New York Times Magazine* about a 59-year-old man who had been in good health, except for a high cholesterol level, for which he took a statin. He complained to his family doctor that he was now out of breath all the time. Even moving about a room caused him to breathe harder. An echocardiogram showed a normal heartbeat, and a stress test did not reveal any reduced blood flow to the heart. But a chest x-ray showed an abnormally light image at the base of each lung. He had no symptoms of pneumonia.

The family doctor referred him to Dr. Charlie Strange, a pulmonologist at the Medical University of South Carolina. The man had never smoked, drank little, and was fairly active. A bronchoscopy found no signs of lung cancer. Dr. Strange tested for interstitial lung disease, of which there are many kinds. But a clue from the bronchoscopy suggested another possibility. The man had a high level of the kind of white blood cell called eosinophils, which often show up in allergic reactions. Dr. Strange wondered if his patient might be allergic to the statin he was taking for his high cholesterol.

After stopping the statin, the man made a rapid recovery. On the first day, it took him a hundred breaths to climb two flights of stairs, and about two weeks later, only eight breaths. Dr. Strange pointed out, however, there was no scientific proof that the statin was responsible.

A study of more than 1,000 users of statins over five years has been completed and its results are planned for publication. The results of the study, funded by the National Institutes of Health, are expected to show a higher rate of cognitive side effects, such as memory problems, than previously reported.

"There are clinicians out there who really are beginning to appreciate that these side effects are substantially more common than one would divine from reading the [medical] literature," Dr. Beatrice A. Golomb, of the University of California at San Diego, and leader of the study, told *The Wall Street Journal*. She added that among patients she has seen outside the study, about 15 percent have developed some cognitive problems connected to their use of statins.

Blood Pressure Once Normal Now Seen as Borderline High

More than 50 million Americans—two-thirds of them over the age of 65—have high blood pressure, or hypertension. Less than 20 million have the condition under control. As part of its effort to reassess this unsatisfactory situation, the federal government's National High Blood Pressure Education Program established a new category, called "prehypertension," in its classification system. The blood pressure in this new category was previously regarded as within the normal range. The change is meant to promote prevention by alerting the 45 million or so Americans (22 percent of adults) that belong in this category of the threat to their health. The other major change in the program guidelines was a recommendation of a low-cost diuretic instead of a more expensive medication in starting drug therapy. But according to a World Health Organization estimate, a big part of the problem is that only half the people who are supposed to be taking a prescription drug for their high blood pressure take it regularly.

I recommend the lifestyle changes suggested in the table below. I also suggest that you check with your doctor whether any over-the-counter or prescription medications you take for other ailments can raise your blood pressure.

Lifestyle Changes to Lower High Blood Pressure

Blood Pressure	Systolic	Diastolic	Action
Stage 2 hypertension	160 or more	100 or more	Lifestyle changes plus treatment with two drugs, one a diuretic
Stage 1 hypertension	140–159	90–99	Lifestyle changes plus a diuretic for most

Lifestyle Changes to Lower High Blood Pressure *(continued)*

Blood Pressure	Systolic	Diastolic	Action
Prehypertension	120–139	80–89	Lifestyle changes consisting of weight loss, more exercise, low-fat diet, more fruit and vegetables, no salt, moderate drinking, no smoking
Normal	Less than 120	Less than 80	No changes needed

Last Word

As you must realize by now, monitoring cholesterol levels for your cardiovascular health is, if anything, more important than ever. What's mostly needed is to look at cholesterol in a different way. You may have to change some of your expectations. For example, your total cholesterol level is not the best measure of heart attack risk. Your triglyceride level must not be dismissed as something of lesser importance. Perhaps most importantly, your LDL cholesterol level is your most reliable gauge to how well you are responding to therapy.

13. Supporting Heart Health with Lifestyle

If you are under the age of 55 and are healthy except for being overweight, try any diet you like for three months or so and see how much weight you lose. Then return to a more balanced diet and keep the weight you lost from coming back. That's the real challenge, because if you go back to your old ways you'll go back to your old weight. To keep that weight from coming back, you need to make a lifestyle change.

Would I recommend a low-carb, high-protein diet? Yes, if you fit the profile described above. If you don't, because of age or risk factors, I think you need to question the wisdom of putting your body under the metabolic stress involved in a radical diet. That is not a yes or no answer, simply a caution. Your doctor will have valuable comments to make. However, if you have any risk factors for heart disease or diabetes other than age and weight, I would recommend against any diet high in saturated fats, even for a period of three months.

Most Americans eat far too much refined grains, sugars, and starches. We also eat too much saturated fat and, even when the food is healthy, too many calories per day. Any lifestyle change that involves permanent weight loss has to involve these three factors.

Ultimately, dieting doesn't work because most people go back to their habitual lifestyles.

Family Values

Childhood habits are hard to break. If you had the good fortune to be raised with healthy eating and exercise habits, you don't have to make the effort that many do who were less fortunate than you. Most parents meant well, but parents then didn't know what we know now. Today people can have the added motivation of wishing to be a good example to their children.

When I see patients in their teens or twenties who are overweight, eat a lot of fast food, smoke, and take little or no exercise, I can guess that their parents look and live the same way. My guess is usually correct. But in such cases, whatever lifestyle changes the young people need to make have to happen in the whole family. Sometimes the whole family goes along with a healthy eating program. Often, some members dig in their heels or treat it as a joke. Then again, in some cases, individuals strike out on their own for a healthy life. The real decision, however, very often lies with the person who buys and prepares the food.

With families, it's never simple. When Alice was 12, she joined a health awareness program at school. In time, she persuaded her father to stop smoking and her mother to serve more vegetables with meals. At 16, much to the surprise and dismay of her parents, Alice herself was smoking cigarettes and eating mostly burgers and pizza. Her parents blamed it on peer pressure. She stopped smoking and got back to healthy eating again, but that was several years later.

Before you make lifestyle changes, you need to consider how they will affect those close to you and how much help or hindrance you can expect to get. Such assistance or opposition is often the deciding factor in whether someone succeeds in making healthy changes or abandons the effort after a short time.

• SONIA AND SODA •

What was I to do about Sonia? She was a very intelligent college student of 20, with a serious weight problem, who drank two or three liters a day of a popular cola. She was very conscious of how quickly she was putting on weight, and she knew all about the health and self-image problems that were likely to ensue. Interestingly, she refused to drink diet cola, although it contained no calories, whereas an 8-ounce glass of regular cola had about 100 calories. (I don't see diet soda as a healthy alternative. It has its own health issues, perhaps chief among them being its acidity. This was presumably not a factor in Sonia's refusal to drink it.)

A can of regular cola contains 140 to 150 calories. If you drank one can a day for a year, you would ingest more than 50,000 calories and add about 15 pounds to your weight. Besides high calorie content, lack of nutritional value, and damage to teeth, soda has another problem. It doesn't satisfy hunger. At Purdue University, fifteen volunteers drank 450 calories of soda every day for four weeks. In another four-week stretch, they ate 450 calories of jelly beans every day. They put on weight in the soda-drinking phase, but not in the jelly bean–eating phase. That was because jelly beans dampened their appetites and they ate less, but soda did not and they ate as much as always.

Why did Sonia drink such huge quantities of cola? Some days, she drank almost 2,000 calories, which approaches the total energy intake recommended for a sedentary adult male. Wouldn't the difference in calories make up for any taste difference between regular and diet colas? But she wouldn't even consider a trial change. I asked her to see a psychiatrist. She agreed, but never went. Last I heard of her, she had returned to school.

Every doctor has difficult patients like Sonia—people smart enough to act responsibly but who behave childishly or perhaps compulsively. If I can figure out what makes them tick, I may be able to help. But if a patient wishes to hide things from a doctor, it's not hard to do. There is usually an emotional component involved. When it comes to food, there often is.

If you need to lose weight, consider how your eating patterns are connected to your emotional ups and downs. It's not necessary to return to childhood incidents and relationships, but simply become aware of any behavioral patterns you have in regard to food. Those close to you may have noticed some, if you have not. Knowing where the emotional pitfalls are located helps you to avoid them.

• • •

Our National Image

After Houston was voted the United States' fattest city by *Men's Fitness* magazine for the third year in a row, Mayor Lee Brown lost 20 pounds by eating less and bicycling more. Governor Bob Taft of Ohio, great-grandson of an American president who weighed more than 300 pounds, works hard at keeping trim and fit. Governor Mike Huckabee of Arkansas, a type 2 diabetic, lost nearly 70 pounds through dieting and exercise. He signed a law banning the sale of soda and snacks in elementary schools and requiring schools to send obesity reports to parents. The governor said he was woken up by a friend's sudden death and a health scare of his own. President Bush is regularly seen running, and he often encourages people to keep fit.

While the United States' weight problem is now very much in the public consciousness, we have yet to see much benefit from it. Federal figures in 2003 showed that obesity rose 61 percent in the United States during the 1990s. About one in three American adults are overweight or obese, with a body mass index of more than 25. (We will look at the body mass index shortly.) Seven out of ten Americans die of chronic diseases for which obesity is a risk factor.

According to the National Center for Health Statistics, the rate of obesity in the United States almost doubled during the 1980s and 1990s.

Age	Obese in 1982	Obese in 1999
50–64	14.4%	26.7%
65–74	12.6%	22.1%
75–84	7.7%	15.1%
85+	4.1%	8.3%

Explanations include the following: farm surpluses kept food prices relatively low; the food industry produced 3,800 calories a day of food for every American; surplus corn was turned into the inexpensive sweetener high-fructose corn syrup; and people who would never think of ordering a second serving were seduced by the fast-food industry into supersize and jumbo helpings. The process is still underway and apparently picking up speed. If you are on the obesity train, the time to get off is now.

Between 1998 and 1999, white Americans had a 7 percent increase in obesity, the largest among any ethnic or racial group. In the year 2000, obesity resulted in 300,000 deaths in the United States and about $117 billion in health-care costs. At $7.7 billion, California spends the most on health care for overweight people. At $87 million, Wyoming spends the least.

The Centers for Disease Control and Prevention reported that almost as many Americans died in 2000 from obesity and inactivity as from tobacco use. Still the leading cause of death, tobacco use claimed 435,000 lives (18.1 percent of those who died). Not far behind, obesity and inactivity cost 400,000 lives (16.6 percent of deaths).

About 129.6 million Americans are overweight or obese—64 percent of the population. One in four is obese. More than 20 percent of American children are overweight or obese.

Are Things Getting Worse?

On any day, almost one in three young people eat fast food, according to a national study of 6,212 children and adolescents by U.S. Department of Agriculture and Harvard Medical School researchers, published in *Pediatrics* in February 2004. The participants who ate fast food consumed an average of 187 more calories that day than those who did not. They ingested 9 more grams of fat, 26 more grams of sugars, and 228 more grams of sugar-sweetened drinks. They consumed less fiber, fruit, non-starchy vegetables, and milk. Not only did the almost one in three young people who ate fast food take in more calories for the day, they took in fewer nutrients.

The city government made a survey of nearly 3,000 children from kindergarten through fifth grade in New York City public schools in May 2003. A startling 43 percent weighed more than their recommended weights, with 19 percent rated as overweight and 24 percent as obese. These results were regarded by health commissioner Thomas R. Frieden as nothing less than a calamity in the making—a future wave of heart disease, diabetes, and other ailments. He told *The New York Times*, "What's changed is the increased sedentary lifestyle, the supersizing fast-food, video game culture, and it's leading to a real epidemic."

Global Bulge

Overseas countries are fast developing problems of their own. "In practically every country on earth there is the most extraordinary escalation in obesity," Dr. Philip James, chairman of the International Obesity Task Force, told the *Times* of London. "But in developing countries it looks like the risk of becoming overweight or obese is even greater because, to put it kindly, people there are born with a biology that expects an inadequate diet. Their bodies are tuned to starvation diets."

Dr. James noted that while there is a global glut of calories, the fat-laden and sugar-rich foods that cause so much obesity are low in nutrients. This means that people can suffer from malnutrition and obesity at the same time. Diabetes and heart disease are other likely consequences.

"Every third death in the world is cardiovascular," Dr. Pekka Puska told the London *Times*. He is director of noncommunicable disease prevention and health promotion at World Health Organization headquarters in Geneva, Switzerland. "Twenty years ago these conditions were diseases of affluence. Only the rich got fat. Now it's the poor who get fat. You get a little bit of development, and urbanization, and the food industry comes in. People consume more and more processed foods, which are high in sugar, fat, and salt. The processed foods are cheap because sugar is cheap and there are lots of subsidized imports of saturated animal fats that are not consumed in the West anymore. It's very dangerous to put my finger on well-known global products, but I'm talking about things like sugary soft drinks and convenience foods."

Pacific Islanders are the fattest people in the world. On some islands, 65 percent of the men and 75 percent of the women are obese. In Britain, one man in seven and one woman in five are obese. Russia and the Czech Republic have much the same high rate. In France, the average woman weighed 4.5 pounds more in 2000 than in 1970, and the average man twice that.

What Is Too Much Weight?

The body mass index (BMI) is the closest that international physicians and researchers have come to agreeing on indicating recommended weights. The BMI balances your weight against your height.

BMI

40 or more	Very severely or morbidly obese
35–39.9	Severely obese
30–34.9	Moderately obese
25–29.9	Overweight
18.5–24.9	Normal range
18.4 or less	Underweight

You can use a chart or calculate your own BMI in several ways. One way is to divide your weight in pounds by your height in inches squared, and multiply the result by 703. Or you can divide your weight in kilograms by your height in meters squared. You can have the CDC calculate your BMI online by going to www.cdc .gov/nccdphp/dnpa/bmi.

However, BMIs don't apply to everyone. If you are an athlete with a large muscle mass, you probably have a high BMI. You can decide for yourself who has a healthy weight among the following. The data are for 2002.

	Height	*Weight*	*BMI*
Sylvester Stallone	5'9"	228	34
Arnold Schwarzenegger	6'2"	257	33
Sammy Sosa	6'0"	220	30
George Clooney	5'11"	211	29
Brad Pitt	6'0"	203	27
Michael Jordan	6'6"	216	25
Venus Williams	6'1"	169	22
Demi Moore	5'5"	130	22
Julia Roberts	5'9"	121	18
Nicole Kidman	5'10"	120	17
Madonna	5'4"	101	17
Gwyneth Paltrow	5'10"	111	16

Apples and Pears

Recently many doctors have been paying more attention to their patients' waistline measurements than to their BMIs. Your waist circumference is an indication of how much visceral or abdominal fat you have. Such fat accumulates, mostly out of sight, around your liver, pancreas, and other internal organs. It causes your middle to bulge in an apple shape. This kind of fat distribution is associated with insulin resistance, type 2 diabetes, the metabolic syndrome, and heart disease. At risk are women with waists of more than 35 inches (88 centimeters) and men with waists of more than 40 inches (100 centimeters).

Fat on the buttocks and thighs, which can result in a pear shape, is formed under the skin and is not regarded as a risk factor for heart disease.

It's not known for sure why central or trunk fat is such a health threat. Many doctors suspect that large fat deposits on or very close to internal organs such as the liver and pancreas may affect how they function. The pancreas secretes insulin, and the liver makes and breaks down blood lipids and numerous proteins, including some with a role in atherosclerosis. A slowing down or speeding up of any of these processes could radically influence how a body functions. Fat cells can secrete substances too. This might be of more importance than previously realized. Many suggestions are being made, but indisputable evidence is hard to find. For example, could excess fat around the liver cause it to manufacture more LDL or less HDL? Doctors who see a lot of patients with excess trunk fat would not be totally amazed to hear that it could.

Lifestyle Changes Need Not Be Painful

Many people, when they hear the term "lifestyle changes," can't help visualizing someone in obvious discomfort. That person may be laboring on a running track, looking at a large plateful of unappetizing greens, or doing something else that he or she clearly finds unenjoyable. Some people enjoy running and eating lots of greens, and I think they would join me in saying, "If you don't like this, do something else." It's really as simple as that. Find healthy food that you *like* to eat, and activities that you *enjoy* doing.

The pleasure principle is very important. If you don't derive pleasure from the food or activity, you probably won't stick with it for very long. We're talking about lifestyle changes here, not ten-day crash diets or makeover programs. I don't want you to live on seaweed and supplements, and exercise till you have to be picked up off the floor. Those kind of programs generate body changes that usually can't be maintained. My approach requires that you stop eating certain unhealthy foods and replace them with equally enjoyable healthy foods. And I want you to get out of your chair or car and do fun things.

There's a lot of confusion at present about whether a low-fat or low-carb diet is best. I belong with those who feel that paying attention to what you eat is what counts. Going on a diet—no matter which one—causes you to look critically at what is on your plate or printed in the menu. We Americans eat too much animal fat and refined carbohydrate. For the sake of our hearts, we need to cut back on both.

Carbs are not inherently bad for us. But because of our lack of activity, we cannot burn up the abundant calories that come in carbs. In addition, many carbs are refined, which means that a lot of their fiber and nutrients have been removed.

The excess weight and consequent health problems so much in the news these days did not come about simply because we're lazy and don't care. These issues go back a long way.

Our Early Ancestors

On cable television, you occasionally see a documentary about some hunter-gatherer group that has survived in a remote place. They are usually nomads who hunt small animals with spears, arrows, or darts and eat whatever berries, fruits, and roots are in season. Honey is their only sugar, and they have to fight bees for that.

From the sparse health information we have about such people, we know that cardiovascular disease is almost unknown among them. Yet they gorge themselves on fatty food when they can find it, holding in the greatest esteem animal parts with the highest fat content.

Wild animals have a low fat content in comparison to domestic animals. For example, in the dry season, African gazelles have a fat content of only 1 to 4 percent, in contrast to the 30 percent or more fat content of the sausages, bacon, and cheese that we eat. Hunter-gatherers crave fats. They are desperate for them! They don't get fats from most berries and fruits. They get some from starchy roots and nuts. Finding enough fat can be a survival problem for people who live as hunter-gatherers. People today are descended from hunter-gatherers, and we have inherited these cravings for edible fats. But our ancestors had to physically exert themselves for fatty food, and we don't.

Presumably you would not survive long as a hunter-gatherer if you were not in excellent health. We might still be living as small groups of very healthy individuals, hunting and gathering, if some of us—thousands of years ago—had not started to farm.

Carb City

In various histories of humankind, you are likely to find the agricultural revolution treated as a great leap forward. But like the industrial revolution that followed millennia later, it had costs as well as benefits. Agriculture permitted people to reside in one place, erect permanent homes, gather possessions, and form an elaborate society. This beat traveling light and moving with the seasons. Towns, and later cities, grew as the population expanded. The population grew because people who would not have survived as hunter-gatherers did survive for longer times in the less challenging environment of early farming communities. They did not survive because of better nutrition. In fact, their nutrition was worse.

Organized growing, harvesting, and storage of cereals meant that people no longer had to search for nuts, berries, fruit, and roots. Domestication of cattle and sheep meant they no longer had to hunt or starve. They now had adequate supplies of grain and fatty meat. These foods were inferior nutritionally to what their hunter-gatherer ancestors ate, but their lower quality was more than compensated for by their reliable availability. People were now less vulnerable to weather and natural disasters. They now ate a high-carb, high-fat diet, but with some important differences from the way we live today. Their carbohydrates came from whole grains. The flesh of domestic animals was consumed mostly on ceremonial occasions—almost certainly not on a daily basis, except perhaps by royalty and warriors. Additionally, people had to till their fields and protect their domestic animals. In other words, they led highly active lives. Yet from the work of archeologists and anthropologists, we know that some of the diseases common today appeared with increasing frequency as these cities grew.

The ancient Greeks had the first health practitioners that we identify as physicians, in that they tried to describe and cure diseases in what we call a scientific way. Their descriptions of disorders—though not their suggested cures—stand up well today. By then, cardiovascular disease was widespread.

Until the industrial revolution in the nineteenth century, dying of hunger remained a realistic concern for people everywhere. When they had to worry about starving to death, food was food, regardless of its nutritional value. Very few people overate or were sedentary on a regular basis. Industry changed that.

In today's so-called postindustrial age, we still have much the same minds and bodies we had thousands of years ago as hunter-gatherers. Theoretically we should evolve at some point into beings that thrive on junk food, soda, and sitting. But evolution is slow. We have left our minds and bodies behind. We still have our fight-or-flight response to perceived threats that causes so much anxiety and stress. And we have our love of fatty food and an instinct to gorge ourselves when the opportunity offers. Most of us no longer bother with whole grains or honey. We have white bread and table sugar, and we drive to the supermarket to obtain them. We have moved, as one researcher memorably put it, "from hunter-gatherer to diabetic couch potato."

Short of hunting and berry gathering, is there anything you can do? Of course. With the wide assortment of foods and recreational facilities available today, you can easily correct the situation. My approach mainly involves avoiding some harmful foods and becoming more active. You'll quickly find that these two things will enrich your life and make you feel better.

We Are Omnivores

Harmful food is a somewhat subjective concept. Food harmful to a 60-year-old sedentary person with insulin resistance may be harmless to a 20-year-old athlete. Leaving aside extremes, nearly all adult Americans need to cut back heavily on animal fats and refined foods of all kinds. In the past couple of decades, we have been joined in this by the populations of other highly developed countries—it's no longer just an American problem. Health problems due to convenient foods too high in fat or sugar are seen as one of the costs of prosperity. They come with the territory, so to speak. We probably can't change the world, but we definitely can protect ourselves and those close to us.

We're not carnivores or herbivores, but omnivores. Teeth tell the whole story. Big cats and other carnivores have long sharp fangs that are ideal for the things we see them do so graphically on TV nature programs. Cows and other herbivores have big flat-crowned teeth to chew the cud. We and other omnivores have a mix of incisors, canines, and molars that permit us to eat almost anything— omnivores, we eat all things. If we wish to or have to, this permits us at one end of the spectrum to live as vegetarians and at the other end to eat high-protein diets. Generally, it's safer in the middle.

In the middle of the spectrum, we eat varied amounts of proteins, fats, and carbohydrates. Many of us, like our hunter-gatherer ancestors, still rely on chance for what we eat! In our case, however, we only rarely have poor hunting days, when all the stores are closed.

I am not a nutritionist or dietician, and I keep my approach to food simplified for use in a doctor's office. That means I have to be careful what I say. My general approach is to eat healthy foods and avoid unhealthy foods. To do that, you have to pay attention to what you eat. Once you pay attention, the rest comes easily.

Proteins and Their Sources

For protein sources, we generally rely on red meat, poultry, and fish. But it's the protein sources rather than the proteins that are desirable or less desirable. Red meat's desirability problem is fairly easily solved by eating only lean meat from which the fat has been trimmed before cooking. Avoid marbled meats, which are impossible to trim, and don't eat red meat in restaurants and other places where you can't trim the fat before it is cooked. Avoid gravy and sauce prepared with fat runoff from meat.

Removing the skin and large, easily identifiable fat pockets from cooked poultry gets rid of a lot of the fat in this excellent protein source.

Fish are tricky. They are a healthy source of protein and un-saturated fats, but also a reservoir of harmful pollutants. They become harmful to eat in three ways. First, herbicides, fungicides, and other chemicals used by farmers drain off the land into rivers and lakes and become lodged in the edible tissues of freshwater fish. Second, pollutants are retained in the edible tissues as bigger fish eat smaller fish, all the way up to the biggest fish at the top of the food chain. Swordfish, king mackerel, and shark can build up dangerous amounts of mercury in their flesh. Third, feeding ground-up fish and animal-derived waste products to farmed fish helps concentrate harmful products in their flesh.

Relatively small ocean fish are presently the safest fish to eat, such as cod, haddock, whiting (hake), pollack, herring, and halibut. Most are caught in deep water far from land, because the more accessible, shallower waters have been overfished and are no longer commercially viable.

Young children, pregnant or nursing women, and women about to become pregnant were found to be most at risk from harmful substances in fish. The American Heart Association recommends that everyone should eat fish at least twice a week. Vulnerable people should avoid swordfish, tuna, and other species with potentially high mercury levels. For most people, the risk involved is far outweighed by the benefits of the protein and omega-3 fatty acids that fish contain.

Fats Come in Threes

Fats in food are almost always a mixture of saturated and unsaturated, the former usually solid at room temperature and the latter usually liquid. The animal fat that you remove from red meat and poultry is mostly saturated fat. Eggs and dairy products have high levels of saturated fat. Tropical oils such as cocoa, coconut, and palm oils are rich in saturated fats, as are macadamia nuts. Experts say that fewer than 20 grams a day are desirable in your diet. I would say a lot fewer. Keep in mind that saturated fats are needed by children (mother's milk is about 45 percent saturated fat).

Unsaturated fats come in two kinds—polyunsaturated and monounsaturated. Some polyunsaturated fats in your food are classified as essential fatty acids—called "essential" because they are essential for bodily function and your body can't manufacture them on its own. Omega-3 and omega-6 fatty acids are polyunsaturated fats. Omega-3 fatty acids are found in coldwater marine fatty fish, in flax, mustard, rape (canola), and hemp seeds, and in walnuts and soybeans. Omega-6 fatty acids are found in pumpkin, flax, sunflower, sesame, hemp, grape, and cotton seeds, and in corn, peanuts, walnuts, soybeans, pecans, almonds, pistachios, wheat germ, rice bran, and safflower.

Oleic acid is the best-known monounsaturated fat. It is found in all vegetable oils. Olive oil, peanut oil, and sesame oil are very rich in it. Avocados and most nuts are also good sources. When you replace saturated fats or carbohydrates in your diet with monounsaturated fats, you lower your LDL.

The National Academy of Sciences guidelines recommend a total fat consumption of 45 to 67 grams in a daily diet of 2,000 calories. Because fat constituents and its food content vary, even among the same foods, you can't be precise in its control. Remember, you almost always find all three fats together. Your best strategy is to replace foods rich in saturated fat with foods rich in unsaturated fat, without counting the grams. This gives you plenty of leeway to enjoy your food and make some permanent changes. Once they have cut back on foods rich in saturated fat for some time, many people remark that its cooking smell and taste become offensive to them.

Fatty Fish

Omega-3 fatty acids have been known for some time to lower the risk of death from heart disease. They reduce triglyceride blood levels, raise HDL, and help get rid of blood clots.

"The higher your blood level of omega-3, the lower your risk," Dr. Christine M. Albert of the Massachusetts General Hospital and Brigham and Women's Hospital in Boston told *The New York Times*. She added, "There isn't any good data on how much fish it takes to get to a certain blood level."

Omega-3 fatty acids are found in fish, seafood, and some vegetable oils, mainly canola, flaxseed, and soybean. But the two most important omega-3 fatty acids—docosahexaenoic acid (DHA) and eicosapentaenoic acid (EPA)—are available mostly in fish. This is why the American Heart Association recommends eating fish at least twice a week. The oils are initially made by algae, which are eaten by small fish, which are in turn eaten by bigger fish. The oils become concentrated in the fish muscle.

In the Harvard nurse study, women who ate fish five times a week had 45 percent less risk of dying of heart disease than women who rarely ate fish. I'm fond of fish, but five times a week might be a little too often, even for me. Those who ate fish two to four times a week had a 30 percent lower risk of nonfatal heart attacks. If you dislike fish, try fish-oil capsules. High-quality fish oils are now available in concentrated form and in different flavors. Make sure the label on the product you use says it has been tested for mercury contamination. To avoid any chance of a fishy odor, do not take more capsules per day than the label recommends.

Grams of Omega-3 Oils per 4-Ounce Serving of Fish or Seafood

2 or More Grams

Pacific herring	2.4	Atlantic salmon	2.1
Atlantic herring	2.3	Sablefish	2.0
Pacific or jack mackerel	2.1		

1–2 Grams

Canned pink salmon	1.9	Coho salmon	1.2
Whitefish	1.9	Bluefish	1.1
Pacific oysters	1.6	Trout	1.1
Pink salmon	1.5	Eastern oysters	1.0
Atlantic mackerel	1.4	Rainbow smelt	1.0
Sockeye or red salmon	1.4	Whiting (hake)	1.0

Less than 1 Gram

Freshwater bass	0.9	Snapper	0.4
Blue mussels	0.9	Sturgeon	0.4
Swordfish	0.9	Atlantic perch	0.3
Rainbow trout	0.8	Fresh or canned clams	0.3
Canned white tuna	0.8	Haddock	0.3
Canned sardines	0.7	Canned light tuna	0.3
Flounder or sole	0.6	Yellowfin tuna	0.3
Halibut	0.5	Atlantic cod	0.2
Rockfish	0.5	Catfish	0.1
Shrimp	0.4		

SOURCE: U.S. Department of Agriculture.

Trans Fats

To give polyunsaturated fats a longer shelf life in stores, manufacturers partially hydrogenate them and process them at high temperatures. The high-temperature processing destroys much of their nutritional value. The hydrogenation has an even more serious effect, giving rise to trans fats. The cis form is the natural form, to which your body is adapted. The trans form is artificially made, is stable, and has a longer shelf life, but it is not accepted by your body as a natural food.

Trans fats are associated with heart disease and cancer. They raise triglyceride and lipoprotein(a) levels in your blood. You can avoid them entirely by not eating fast food and reading nutrition labels on food packages. Manufacturers are required by law to list trans fat content. Any food that is partially hydrogenated or contains vegetable shortening or margarine contains trans fats.

Carbs to Think About

For many years, interest in the deleterious effects of dietary fats on blood cholesterol overwhelmed attention to how carbohydrates affect blood sugar and insulin. Things have changed, with a vengeance. The federal Institute of Medicine, the authority that sets the recommended daily intake of nutrients, set 130 grams of carbohydrate as the recommended minimum daily intake for adults and children. Most Americans eat more than this minimum amount. In general, men eat 200 to 330 grams a day, and women eat 180 to 230 grams. In the first stage of one popular low-carb diet, you are asked to eat no more than 20 grams of carbohydrate a day. An 8-ounce glass of orange juice or a typical potato contains 26 grams of carbohydrate.

Most of us have heard by now that the carbohydrates we eat are broken down into glucose that is transported in our bloodstreams. The hormone insulin, secreted by the pancreas in response to rising blood sugar, regulates what happens to the glucose. The muscles and liver use much of it as fuel. Some of the

Are You Insulin-Resistant?

Insulin resistance is hard to diagnose. There are no tests for it that can be conveniently performed in a doctor's office, and you can have a normal level of blood glucose and be insulin-resistant. An experienced doctor, however, can recognize its signs. A high insulin level and trouble losing weight are often signs. Excess weight increases insulin resistance, often leading to impaired glucose tolerance and, ultimately, type 2 diabetes.

excess glucose is stored by insulin as a fuel reserve in the form of fat. The fat will be burned as fuel when the insulin level is low.

The problems with carbohydrates begin when you put on too much weight. The fatter you get, the more insulin your pancreas secretes into your bloodstream with each meal. If you also have an inherited tendency to be insulin-resistant—your cells become less sensitive to insulin—higher blood levels of insulin become necessary to control your blood sugar. It's debatable whether excess weight or insulin resistance is the original cause. As you continue to gain weight, your elevated insulin level makes it easier for you to store your blood glucose as fat and harder for you to burn it as fuel.

As the insulin levels of healthy people rise in response to the food they eat, their appetites become suppressed. They stop eating and don't put on excess weight. Their blood sugar levels remain more or less stable. But the high insulin levels of overweight, insulin-resistant people burn up their blood sugar, making them ravenously hungry as their bodies run out of fuel. This is why you can be hungry again soon after a large carbohydrate-rich meal.

In healthy as well as insulin-resistant people, carbohydrates in the form of refined grains, starches, and sugars are quickly converted to glucose and are carried into the blood. They cause a spike in the blood sugar level and an answering surge of insulin.

Even after using some glucose as fuel and storing some as fat, the insulin level remains sufficiently high to cause a drop in the blood sugar level. You feel hungry and crave carbohydrates. You eat more carbohydrates. The whole cycle begins again. Green, leafy vegetables are good carbs, as indeed are most nonstarchy vegetables.

The carbohydrates of nonstarchy vegetables are digested more slowly and don't cause a spike in the blood sugar level. These are the so-called good carbs. You can eat lots of them without putting on extra weight.

Fruit is a matter of sugar content. Eat more of the less sweet, and less of the more sweet. Raw, unprocessed fruits are healthy in reasonable quantity. Commercial fruit juices and bottled, canned, or otherwise processed fruits may not be.

Fresh vegetables and raw fruit contain all kinds of micronutrients, known and unknown, that give us good health and enjoyment in life. To exclude them permanently from your daily diet is not a wise decision.

A Carb Worth Seeking: Fiber

Eating food with a high fiber content makes you satiated more quickly, so that you eat less, consume fewer calories, and put on less weight. A diet high in fiber lowers your risk for heart disease and diabetes. But most Americans eat less than half the amount of fiber that they need. Many eat only 8 to 10 grams per day. The following is the generally recommended intake:

	Women	Men
19–50 years	25 grams	38 grams
Over 50	21 grams	30 grams

How many calories does fiber contain? While fats contain 9 calories per gram, fiber contains 1.5 to 2.5 calories per gram. Protein and other carbohydrates have 4 calories per gram. But many nutritionists count the calorie content of fiber as zero. This is because much fiber is insoluble and therefore indigestible. Soluble fiber is partially digested and yields calories. These calories are offset by the calories lost in fats trapped by fiber and transported undigested out of the body. In addition, soluble fiber lowers cholesterol. Such estimates can become complicated. For most people, though, any calorie intake from fiber is likely to be so low as to be not worth counting.

Your digestive system evolved to consume high-fiber foods. They are what your body needs. Fiber, along with various nutrients, is often lost in processed foods. Some is removed, and some is destroyed in high-temperature processing. This loss of fiber helps increase the impact of processed foods and refined grains on your blood sugar and insulin levels.

Whole grains, fruit, and vegetables are the natural sources of fiber. A lot of fiber is contained in the skin, so don't peel when you don't have to. If you think that your low-carb diet may not be providing you with sufficient fiber, you should change your diet so that it does. If you don't add fresh fruit and vegetables to your diet, take a commercial fiber preparation.

However, healthy people eat fresh fruit and vegetables. Your body needs their vitamins, minerals, and micronutrients, as well as their fiber.

I recommend soluble fiber for cholesterol reduction. While fiber also helps diabetics control their blood sugar, such large daily amounts are needed—about 50 grams—that it's often not practical. Because the Western diet rarely supplies sufficient fiber, I recommend that you take soluble fiber in the form of a powder supplement to reduce cholesterol and help lower blood sugar.

High-Fructose Corn Syrup

In reducing the fat content of food, processors found that it lost taste. They discovered that they could restore a pleasing taste by adding sugars. Sprinkling the food with table sugar was no longer an option with health-conscious buyers. Sucrose, fructose, and glucose were added to the food in invisible form. High-fructose corn syrup is perhaps the most widely used commercial sweetener. This is not the same corn syrup used for pouring on pancakes. It is sweeter than table sugar and about 20 percent cheaper. Virtually all commercially baked cakes, pies, and pastries are loaded with it and other sugars and sweeteners under various names. These are not the only foods that make use of high-fructose corn syrup. It's frequently used in some brands of pizza, beer, ketchup, cookies, and yogurt, to name only a few.

"I think it's a huge problem," Dr. Richard Anderson of the federal Human Nutrition Research Center in Beltsville, Maryland, told the *AARP Bulletin*. "High-fructose corn syrup is metabolized differently than other sugars, and it has a different effect on health."

Avoiding packaged baked goods is a good way to start ridding yourself of these hidden sugars and sweeteners.

Some Internet Sources of Nutrition Advice

- American Dietetic Association, www.eatright.org. Click on "Food & Nutrition Information."
- Center for Science in the Public Interest, www.cspinet.org.
- HealthAtoZ, www.healthatoz.com. Click on the consumer health site, then "Lifestyles," and then "Nutrition."

• U.S. Department of Agriculture, www.usda.gov/fnutrition.html.

Making Use of the Glycemic Index

Following a low-carb diet for the short term in order to lose excess weight is one thing. Cutting back on your carbohydrate intake as a long-term lifestyle change is another. Cutting back on refined grains, starchy vegetables, and sugars in your daily food will make a big difference. Notice that I usually say *cutting back* or *reducing* instead of *eliminating*. That's because it's almost impossible to eliminate saturated fats and sugars from American foods. Trying to is not worth the aggravation. Besides, if you set your aim too high, you are raising the likelihood of quitting due to frustration.

Many carbohydrates baffle people. They have no notion of whether some particular food is healthy or not. Even people who are relatively knowledgeable can be surprised by how little or how much some carbs affect blood sugar. Seeing the glycemic index for the first time is almost certain to deliver some surprises.

The glycemic index ranks carbohydrate foods according to their impact on blood sugar and insulin levels. The longer it takes a food to be digested, the lower its impact. Fats in food slow the body's absorption and thereby lower a food's glycemic index. Sugars, starches, and refined grains tend to have the highest scores because they are digested most quickly and cause a spike in the blood sugar level. The fiber in green vegetables, beans, and whole grains slows down their digestion. The protein and fat contents of foods slow their digestion.

The glycemic index numbers for fresh and commercially

prepared fruit juices may be quite different. Commercial processing very often removes pulp and fiber, increasing the juice's absorbability by the body and thereby raising its glycemic index.

Low-glycemic diets are increasingly popular. However, what you have to watch for is that the glycemic index does not take calories into consideration. Foods low on the glycemic index may not cause a spike in your blood sugar level, but that does not mean you should eat larger helpings of them. Eat a lot of the ones rich in calories and you will put on weight.

You don't have to go on a low-glycemic diet to benefit from the glycemic index. You can use an expanded version of the sample given here to check your favorite foods and even brands.

A Short Version of the Glycemic Index

High GI (above 70)

Tofu frozen dessert	115	French fries	75
Maltose	105	Graham crackers	74
Dates	103	Saltine crackers	74
Parsnip	97	Bagel	72
Baguette	95	Corn chips	72
Pretzel	83	Soda crackers	72
Jelly beans	80	Watermelon	72
Rice cakes	80	Millet	71
Doughnut	76		

Intermediate GI (55–70)

White bread	70	Cantaloupe	65
Cornmeal	68	Cola	65
Rye crackers	68	Couscous	65
Croissant	67	Black bean soup	64
Green pea soup	66	Canned beets	64
Pineapple	66	Raisins	64
Split pea soup with ham	66	Rye bread	64

Intermediate GI (55–70) *(continued)*

Shortbread cookie	64	Papaya	58
Table sugar	64	Pear	58
Honey	62	Apricot	57
Hamburger bun	61	Pita	57
Pizza	60	Banana	56
Vanilla ice cream	60	Corn	56
Blueberry muffin	59	Potato chips	56
Basmati white rice	58	Mango	55

Low GI (below 55)

Muesli	54	Baked beans	44
Oat and raisin muffin	54	Cinnamon muffin	44
Pound cake	54	Custard	43
Sourdough bread	54	Orange	43
Yam	54	Peach	42
Canned kidney beans	52	Apple juice	40
Kiwi	52	Pinto beans	39
Strawberry preserves	51	Plum	39
Cheese tortellini	50	Navy beans	38
Linguini	50	Apple	38
Vanilla ice milk	50	Tomato soup	38
Carrots	49	Fruit yogurt	36
Milk chocolate	49	Chocolate milk	35
Pumpernickel bread	49	Vermicelli	35
Bulgur	48	Garbanzo beans	34
Grapefruit juice	48	Butter beans	33
Oatmeal	48	Spaghetti	33
Peas	48	Fettucini	32
Frozen green peas	47	Lima beans	32
Grapes	46	Skim milk	32
Macaroni	46	Cannellini beans	31
Fresh orange juice	46	Soy milk	31
Fresh pineapple juice	46	Black beans	30
Apple muffin	44	Green or brown lentils	30

Low GI (below 55) (continued)

Whole milk	30	Cherries	22
Kidney beans	29	Fructose	22
Red lentils	27	Soy beans, boiled	16
Barley	25	Prunes	15
Grapefruit	25	Plain yogurt	14

Shedding Excess Weight

Excess weight is usually a consequence of unhealthy eating habits and inactivity. When I talk about losing excess weight, I am talking, of course, about body fat. You never want to lose so much

How Much Is Body Fat?

When you diet and exercise, you lose fat and build muscle. Stepping on a scale won't tell you how much of one you have lost and of the other gained. For example, the scale indicates that you have lost 10 pounds in body weight. This could represent a loss of 13 pounds of fat and a gain of 3 pounds of muscle. In this case, the positive change is far more than the scale indicates.

It's hard to tell how much fat you have lost because it's hard to reliably measure the percentage of fat in your body. Underwater weighing is the most accurate, if least convenient, method. Measurement with a special skinfold caliper can be done at home, but you must allow for a 5 percent margin of error. Bioelectric impedance can have an even larger margin of error.

The body fat percentage is usually more than 20 percent for overweight men and more than 30 percent for overweight women. When a woman's body fat drops below 16 percent, her periods may become irregular and she may suffer bone loss and become vulnerable to fractures.

as an ounce of muscle tissue. A 350-pound wrestler with 5 to 7 percent body fat might not have a single pound of excess weight. Appearances can be deceptive. A wiry person may not qualify for a bodybuilding contest and yet have a high lean-to-fat ratio and be very healthy. But not all thin people are healthy. A very thin person may not have much fat but not much muscle tissue either. Such a person's lean-to-fat ratio can be unhealthily low.

Loss of muscle tissue is one of the characteristics of aging. People who make no effort to maintain their muscles develop skinny arms and legs as they get older. If they also put on weight in their midsection, that and skinny limbs can make them look older than they actually are.

We have already discussed how excess weight around the middle—apple shape—is connected to insulin resistance and, through that, to both heart disease and type 2 diabetes.

Burning Calories

By weight, fat in food has more than twice as many calories as carbs and protein in food. Calories measure energy. Thus, it requires more than twice as much activity to use up a gram of food fat than a gram of carbohydrate or protein. A reasonably active person burns 2,000 calories a day just for body maintenance. If your calorie intake exceeds your body requirement, you put on weight.

Fat	1 gram = 9 calories
Carbohydrate	1 gram = 4 calories
Protein	1 gram = 4 calories

To lose a pound in weight, you must get rid of about 3,500 calories. You can either burn those calories in exercise or not ingest them in the first place. If you reduced your food intake by 500 calories a day for seven days, you would lose that pound. If your daily intake is 3,000 rather than 2,000 calories, the reduction may not be hard to do. Dropping that muffin, doughnut, or pastry from your daily menu may be sufficient.

Why not count carbs and forget about calories, as some diets recommend? Counting carbs is counting calories by another name. It amounts to the same thing. Baked goods, french fries, and other carbohydrate-rich foods are very high in calories. Eliminating them from your diet gets rid of important calorie sources, which is what leads some experts to claim that low-carb, high-protein diets, like all other diets, achieve weight loss solely through calorie reduction. However, the high fat content of the food you eat helps keep you satiated longer.

Athletes and people who do strenuous physical work burn the large amounts of calories they often ingest. But you can't depend on exercise to consume the excess calories you take in. It's usually too hard to do. The human body evolved to maintain a constant weight during times of scarcity and plenty. When you burn calories through exercise, you feel hunger pangs—your body is telling you to restore the lost calories through eating more food. Assuming that you don't give in and continue to burn calories, your body tries to conserve energy and protect itself against further calorie loss. One way it does this is by becoming more efficient. The mile you ran a few days ago burned 100 calories. Today it burns only 90.

Another difficulty is the unbalanced equation between calories in and calories out. It takes a lot of exercise to burn calories and only very little food to replace them. For example, the 300 calories you burned in a 45-minute run can be replaced with two apples or just one cookie.

Consider if eating 2,000 calories and burning 800 calories

through exercise each day is the same as eating 1,200 calories and not exercising. You might burn 800 calories a day by running hard for two hours, but you are going to be very hungry all the time if you are doing that and eating only 2,000 calories a day. Your friends may not find you much fun to be around! Of course, they also may not find you very pleasant if you are eating only 1,200 calories a day. But of these two extremes, I think cutting back on calories is more efficient and comfortable than burning them in quantity.

Exercise helps your body to function better, builds muscles, and helps prevent weight gain. Weight loss, however, is much more easily achieved through diet. It doesn't sound easy, and it wouldn't be easy if you were consuming only 2,000 calories a day. Many of us consume twice that amount and still imagine we have a reasonably healthy diet. Try cutting back on saturated fats and refined grains and sugars. That alone cuts many people's calorie intake in half.

A combination of diet and moderate exercise is the best approach. Exercise builds lean muscle, which has a higher metabolic rate and burns more calories.

Some Weight Control Hints

Here are some things that my patients and I have found helpful in controlling weight.

Record what you eat. Keep a record of how much you eat and drink and how much exercise you engage in. You may be surprised by how much you eat and how little you exercise. Many people who think of themselves as eating little and always on the go wonder why they don't lose weight. They usually remember half the amount they eat and double the amount they exercise. They are not lying. They are just fooling themselves.

Look at what's on your plate. Before reaching for your fork, check out your food. If you don't know what it is because it's smothered in gravy, politely investigate.

Judge the portion size. Is this more than you normally eat? When a restaurant with a popular baked ziti dish increased its size by 50 percent for some regular customers, they all ate the extra food without noticing. Vigilance counts. And so does eating 50 percent more food.

Count calories in real life? Making educated guesses about refined carbs, sugar, and saturated fat can be hard enough. Most people's food would be cold by the time they did the calculations. For a healthy lifestyle, you make guesses all the time, accepting that some of them will be wrong. But for a short-term weight loss diet, you need to be fairly exact about the number of calories you consume. This is one of the few times I recommend processed foods. Reading the package labels enables you to accurately add up the calories.

On a diet, keep the food variety down. You are more easily satiated when the food is monotonous and dull. Variety stimulates your appetite. This is why people, after a big meal, can still find room for a delicious-looking dessert. On the other hand, people quit diets because the food is so boring.

Avoid a refined-grain breakfast. First of all, of course, eat breakfast. To keep your blood sugar at a steady level, you need to eat at the beginning of the day. People who have cut refined grains out of other meals often make an exception for breakfast. But muffins, doughnuts, or toast don't satisfy your needs for long. In fact, many people find that they eat more in the course of a day after a refined-carb breakfast such as a muffin. Breakfasts of eggs, yogurt, fruit, or high-fiber cereals satisfy food cravings much longer.

Why Not Simply Suction Away the Fat?

Why should people deprive themselves of eating fatty meat and sugary pastry, or hours of watching TV while drinking beer, when they can have their excess fat removed by liposuction? It's a reasonable question, and one which until recently doctors could not answer with certainty. In fact, some plastic surgeons have recommended liposuction as a healthy solution to excess fat.

In liposuction, surgeons break up adipose tissue beneath the skin and suction off the fatty cells. With almost 385,000 procedures a year, this is the most frequently performed kind of cosmetic surgery in the United States. Most of the people who have the procedure are women aged 19 through 50.

An authoritative study, published in the *New England Journal of Medicine* on June 17, 2004, showed that liposuction does not reduce risk factors for heart disease and diabetes. Its results look good in a mirror but not in blood tests in a medical lab. If you have liposuction, you will look better, but don't expect to see improvements in your cholesterol, triglyceride, glucose, insulin, and blood pressure levels.

This finding surprised the researchers who conducted the study, at the Center for Human Nutrition at the Washington University School of Medicine in St. Louis. They expected to show that fat removal by liposuction lowers cardiac risk. In the study, about 20 pounds of fat was removed from under the skin of fifteen abdominally obese women in their forties. Seven had type 2 diabetes. This amount of fat, nearly one-fifth of their total body fat, is four times the amount normally removed in a liposuction. Such large-volume liposuctions, however, are becoming more frequent. Ten to twelve weeks after the procedure, the women looked healthier and the researchers expected this to be confirmed by lab tests on their blood samples. The results showed no improvements.

The lead researcher, Dr. Samuel Klein, said that this study should end the debate about what liposuction could achieve, because it was more carefully prepared and conducted than earlier studies. In studies that had previously found benefits from liposuction, Dr. Klein said that after liposuction the participants may have started dieting and exercising and the benefits came from these rather than the liposuction. The women in his study, he said, promised not to begin any diet or exercise program after liposuction. Although the participants were all women, Dr. Klein believed that the study results applied equally to men.

The fact that liposuction did not show any metabolic improvement or reduction of risk factors for heart disease and diabetes did not surprise Dr. Philipp Scherer of the Albert Einstein College of Medicine in New York. He said that liposuction removed fat from beneath the skin, but not visceral fat—the fat around the liver and other organs that is associated with high blood lipids, elevated glucose, and inflammation.

"Unfortunately, these visceral fat pads cannot be targeted by simple liposuction," Dr. Scherer told *The New York Times*. He added that visceral fat deposits are not inert but act like endocrine organs, secreting hormones and other substances into the blood. These secretions may cause inflammation and play other roles in the atherosclerosis process. They may also travel directly to the liver and interfere with its regulation of cholesterol and glucose.

The bodies of obese people contain at least 80 billion to 120 billion fat cells. Those of lean people contain about 40 billion. Additionally, most of the fat cells of obese people are larger in size than those of lean people. The larger fat cells are more metabolically active and likely to secrete harmful substances. Weight loss, regardless of how it is achieved, results from a reduction in both the size and the number of fat cells. An active lifestyle and healthy eating beat any quick fix, including liposuction.

A surefire way to measure how your healthier lifestyle is benefiting your body is to follow the progress of your LDL cholesterol level. As they get fitter, most people notice a drop in their LDL levels, even those whose level was already in the desirable range.

Foods to Lower Your LDL

LDL cholesterol plays an important role in arterial wall inflammation. By lowering the amount of LDL in your bloodstream, you may lessen the inflammation. At the very least, you do not encourage it to progress further. No evidence exists that a lowering of your LDL level results in a lowering of your C-reactive protein or fibrinogen levels, but it would not be unreasonable to expect this to happen since those levels are responsive to inflammation.

We know that many doctors consider the normal ranges for cholesterol to be too high, including that for LDL. (The LDL normal range for a healthy person is less than 130. For someone with heart disease, diabetes, or multiple cardiac risk factors, it is less than 100.) Even if your LDL is within the normal range, it could benefit you to lower it. Of course, it would not make sense to take a drug to do it. But if you could lower your LDL by eating cholesterol-lowering foods, it would certainly be worth doing.

Can diet alone, without drugs, lower your LDL by a significant amount? In my practice, I have certainly seen patients lower their LDL levels by 25 to 30 percent through food alone and no drugs. This was put to the test by a team led by Dr. David J. A. Jenkins, professor of nutritional sciences at St. Michael's Hospital of the University of Toronto. They put forty-six healthy adults on three diets. The first was a vegetarian diet low in saturated fats. The second was this same low-fat vegetarian diet supplemented by a statin (a lovastatin, one of several different kinds of statin on the market). The third was a fiber-rich vegetarian diet made up of food known to lower cholesterol. The participants were randomly assigned to one of the three diets, and they ate it for a month.

At the start of the test, the participants had total cholesterol levels of 250 to 260 and LDL levels above 160. Those on the low-fat vegetarian diet lowered their LDL levels by 8 percent. Those on the low-fat vegetarian diet plus a statin lowered theirs by 30.9 percent. The third group, on the fiber-rich vegetarian diet of cholesterol-lowering foods, reduced their LDL levels by

28.6 percent. The percentage difference between the group taking a statin and that taking cholesterol-lowering foods was so small, it's fair to say that diet can take the place of drugs in lowering LDL.

The catch is that many people would find the diet of cholesterol-lowering foods too spartan to stay on for any length of time. It's not known how long the benefits of the diet lasted after it was abandoned. Here's what they ate each day.

Breakfast

Hot oat-bran cereal, with sugar and psyllium (as Metamucil)
Soy milk
Strawberries
Oat-bran bread
Plant-sterol margarine substitute (no-trans-fat variety)
Jam

Snack

Almonds
Fresh fruit
Soy milk

Lunch

Spicy black bean soup
Sandwich of sliced soy, tomato, cucumber, and lettuce, with plant-sterol margarine substitute, on oat-bran bread

Snack

Almonds
Psyllium
Fresh fruit

Dinner

Tofu with ratatouille
Pearled barley
Vegetables

Snack

Psyllium
Fresh fruit
Soy milk

Foods to Raise Your HDL

Intense aerobic exercise, quitting smoking, and anticholesterol drugs frequently cause a rise in HDL. A less spectacular but very dependable HDL rise can be achieved through weight loss. For every 7 pounds of body weight lost, your HDL level rises by 1, according to Dr. Michael Miller, director of the Center for Preventive Cardiology at the University of Maryland Medical Center. The only difficulty is that some weight-loss diets lower all your blood lipid levels, including your HDL.

• Most people who have heart attacks have an HDL level below 40. An increase of 1 percent in HDL has been linked to a

2 to 3 percent decrease in heart attacks. Having an HDL level above 40 is desirable, but some doctors believe that it should be above 60 to deliver significant benefits. You also need to consider the ratio between your total cholesterol level and HDL cholesterol level (that is, total cholesterol divided by HDL). In the Framingham Heart Study, people with a cholesterol/HDL ratio of 3 to 1 or lower were least likely to have heart attacks. The average ratio for Americans is 4.5 to 1. For people with heart disease, it is often 5.5 to 1. Needless to add, the higher your total cholesterol, the higher your HDL must be for a healthy ratio.

How can you lower your weight but not your HDL? If you go on a low-fat diet that replaces the fats with carbohydrates without also reducing the calories consumed, you could lower your HDL by as much as 20 percent, Dr. Miller told *The New York Times*. Additionally, when more than 60 percent of the calories in your diet come from carbohydrates, your triglyceride level rises. This happens even when the carbohydrates are whole grains.

Monounsaturated fats boost the HDL level. Use them to replace saturated fats and refined carbohydrates. (Replacing saturated fats with polyunsaturated fats brings down all blood lipid levels, including HDL.) But all these intricate arrangements have already been made for you in a diet that has been around for more than two thousand years, the Mediterranean-style diet. Accompanying the food with two glasses of wine helps raise your HDL even further.

Some believe that red wine is more effective than white because it contains more of certain ingredients. Others say that these ingredients matter less than the easing of stress, and thus all alcohol in moderation is more or less equally effective.

Foods to Lower Your Blood Pressure

The DASH (Dietary Approaches to Stop Hypertension) diet from the National Institutes of Health has been around for some years now. It has enabled many people with slightly elevated blood pressure (mild hypertension) to use diet instead of drugs to return to the normal range. The diet depends on cutting back on salt and eating plenty of vegetables and fruits rich in potassium, magnesium, and fiber. Potassium may be the most important ingredient—it helps the body rid itself of excess sodium and water. The following are examples:

Apricots	Grapes	Prunes
Artichokes	Kale	Raisins
Bananas	Mangoes	Spinach
Beans	Melons	Squash
Broccoli	Orange juice	Strawberries
Carrots	Oranges	Sweet potatoes
Collards	Peaches	Tangerines
Dates	Peas	Tomatoes
Grapefruit	Pineapple	Turnip greens
Grapefruit juice	Potatoes	

To Walk or Not to Walk

In his report *Physical Activity and Health*, the surgeon general advises "people of all ages to include a minimum of thirty minutes of physical activity of moderate intensity (such as brisk walking) on most, if not all, days of the week." Thirty minutes! Every day!

Physical activity of moderate intensity is anything that makes your heart beat at a rate equivalent to walking at 3 or 4 miles per hour. The Centers for Disease Control and Prevention conducted a survey in 2001 to see how much of this kind of activity was going on. A quarter of the people who responded denied any moderate activity at all. Another quarter did not meet the surgeon general's requirements. For the same year, the average American over age 15 spent more than an hour a day behind a car steering wheel, according to the Federal Highway Administration. Federal health agencies used to inquire about how much time Americans spent in gyms or playing ball. Nowadays they ask if we do anything at all.

It would take you about twenty minutes to walk a mile at 3 miles per hour. You would burn about 100 calories. If you walked a mile every day of the week, you would burn 700 calories. You need to burn 3,500 calories to lose a pound of weight. Therefore you would lose 1 pound every five weeks of daily walking, and more than 10 pounds in a year.

By attaching step counters to the legs of a thousand volunteers, University of Colorado researchers estimated that the average person takes about 5,900 steps a day, which is equivalent of about 3 miles. If they took an extra 2,000 steps, about another mile, most people would lose another 100 to 150 calories each day. This would mean a loss of more than 10 pounds a year. The researchers found that participants were amazed at how few steps they took and at how fast they lost weight when they started deliberate walking.

I should add that the surgeon general continued, after the quote above, by saying, "For most people, greater health benefits can be obtained by engaging in physical activity of more vigorous intensity or of longer duration."

A 150-pound person doing these activities for thirty minutes would burn about this number of calories:

Activity	Calories Burned	Activity	Calories Burned
Jogging	338	Walking briskly	150
Climbing stairs	306	Supermarket shopping	122
Tennis	275	Cleaning house	122
Carrying a heavy load	273	Sweeping the floor	85
Lifting weights	234	Dusting	80
Cycling on level ground	221	Ironing	77
Shoveling snow	205	Preparing a meal	74
Low-impact aerobics	171	Desk work	51
Gardening	170	Watching television	36

Daily Walking

Walk briskly for at least thirty minutes each day. Doing this helps keep your cardiovascular system healthy. This will probably be enough exercise to keep you from putting on more weight, but probably not enough to cause you to lose any. You don't need much exercise to keep heart disease and diabetes at bay—or even to alleviate a cardiac or diabetic condition. But you need to be active almost every day.

Some of us are "weekend warriors," getting lots of exercise on the weekend but not much during the week. This exercise is equally beneficial to that done in smaller amounts every day. The main drawback is that sedentary people who overexert themselves on occasion are more liable to injure themselves than people who keep their bodies supple with daily exercise and have no reason to engage in anything overly strenuous.

Taking a half-hour walk each day doesn't sound like much of an exercise commitment. But if it's truly a *commitment* on your part, you may find that it's not quite as easy as it appears.

Mary Jo, for instance, began each day fully intending to walk. But things kept cropping up and she seemed to be always too busy to take a break. Usually by the time she got a chance to walk, it was too late to go. This seemed to happen on most days of the week.

"Are these things that crop up important?" I asked.

"You think I should give my walk more priority?" Mary Jo responded. "I will."

That's one thing to keep in mind. Give your daily walk high priority. You rarely get around to doing the things near the bottom of your to-do list.

But it's not always easy to give your daily walk high priority, especially where family is concerned. Liz spent just about every waking minute taking care of her children and working full-time. She drove the kids to school before work and picked them up afterward. Although she was always on the go, her work and driving were sedentary. Apart from housework, she had little sustained physical activity. How could she walk when she had no time to herself? Her eldest daughter provided the answer. She rearranged the kids' day so that their mother had time to walk. When Liz forgot, the kids reminded her. Once in a while, they even came along with her.

You too can make your daily walk something that your family and friends expect of you. But don't wait for one of your children to arrange it.

Harry's problem was where he lived. Walking on local roads was risky because of high-speed traffic and lack of sidewalks. He took to stopping at a small state park on his way home from work. It was a little out of his way, but instead of hindering him, the extra effort required reinforced his commitment to daily walking. This was something that he did every weekday, and anything that interrupted it needed to be important.

The places where you walk need to be suitable for brisk, uninterrupted walking. Strolling in a shopping mall and looking in every other store window is less than ideal. The same holds for places where you are likely to bump into acquaintances and stop for a chat.

National park rangers check out climbers for safety on the lower slopes of Mount Rainier, the 14,410-foot volcanic peak that looms above Seattle. Regularly, properly equipped climbers fall or are trapped in sudden, unpredictable storms. The rangers turn back many people wearing T-shirts and shorts and sometimes even stiletto heels. For walking, you don't need any special clothing or equipment. A good pair of walking shoes, however, will be easier on your feet, especially if you are a diabetic. Loose clothing will be more comfortable.

You may need to allow for extremes of heat and cold. In hot weather, early-morning or late-evening walks may be pleasant. For really hot spells, an indoor track or swimming pool can be an attractive alternative. Wearing adequate clothing usually provides for cold weather.

Michael bought three books on walking, some brightly colored outfits, and several pairs of special shoes. He was continuing research on the project, but he hadn't actually done any walking yet! I suggested that he might be causing delay by overpreparing for the event—after all, he was not climbing Everest. But he was adamant. Before he went walking, he needed to complete his planning and get things in order. I see dozens of Michaels in city parks—people with expensive outfits, bikes, or whatnot. Mostly, they are standing around looking pleased with themselves rather than exercising. At least they are not home sitting in front of the television.

Off the Couch and on the Move

- Give your daily walk high priority. Record a time for it in your daily planner.

- Make your daily walk something that your family and friends expect of you.
- Choose places suitable for safe, brisk, uninterrupted walking.
- You don't need special footwear or clothing.
- Make allowances for heat and cold, and dress appropriately.
- Don't delay by overpreparing for the event.

Increasing Fitness

Walking for thirty minutes a day is the *minimum* requirement for an active lifestyle. It will help keep your joints from stiffening, which is often the most visible sign of aging. If you are reasonably fit, daily walking will help keep you that way. But if you have let your body go, daily walking will probably not be enough to get it back in shape, even with a healthy diet.

As we discussed before, diet is a more efficient way to lose fat than exercise—although a combination of both is best. When thinking about exercise, it's not a bad idea to forget about losing fat altogether. Instead, think about building muscle. For every two pounds of muscle you build on your body, you burn an extra 20 to 30 calories a day.

Muscle loss is one of the problems of putting on weight and getting older. Heavier people move about less energetically and some of their muscle tissue atrophies for lack of use. Loss of muscle tissue causes the bony look of many old people who are healthily lean. Use it or lose it. Moderate exercise helps prevent muscle loss and maintains strength.

Not long ago, in a fitness book, I noticed a list of a hundred things that exercise can do for you. You know the kind of things.

You can eat more without gaining weight. You have more energy. You feel better about yourself. You feel younger. You look younger. With a few unimportant modifications, I agreed with all one hundred and had another twenty or so of my own to add.

One important benefit of exercise is not itself visible in the mirror but helps account for any bodily enhancement that you see there. Exercise contributes in a big way to metabolic balance. Having your systems and organs in working balance is what gives you a healthy, wholesome appearance. Along with feeling affection for other people, much of the joy of life comes from a simple pleasure of existence, which is physical as well as spiritual.

How Should You Work Out?
And How Intensely?

What should you do to work out? First of all, find something you enjoy doing. If it gets boring, switch to something else. Avoid all "no pain, no gain" routines and most things that are high-impact or can easily result in injury. The physical demands of the exercise should not be above what you can presently manage without great discomfort. Swimming is the one exercise that I recommend to everyone, almost regardless of their state of health. Start out modestly with everything else. Ask advice from knowledgeable people. They are usually happy to give it. Keep in mind that bicycling and skating can result in injuries and may not be the best things to try first.

How intensely should you exercise? You do not want to cross your anaerobic threshold, the point where you switch from burning fat to burning sugar. This can happen when you exercise too hard. People who become fixated on exercise can end up in their sugar-burning zone. If they exercised *less* intensely, they would be more likely to lose weight and less likely to get injured. To lose weight, you need to burn fat.

To find your maximum workload, you need to take a metabolic stress test. The metabolic stress test catches people who are exercising too much or too intensely. I use the metabolic stress test to help people learn where their optimum fat-burning zone is. In this way, they can adjust their exercise to burn as much fat as possible. The metabolic stress test is the only way to discover when you are burning the most fat as you exercise. This test used to be expensive. Now it is more affordable and more available.

If a metabolic stress test is not available, you can do what many experts recommend by exerting yourself in a target range from 50 to 85 percent of your *maximum* heart rate. This, of course, is only a "guesstimate" of what your heart rate should be for an optimally beneficial workout. Your heart rate, or pulse, is the number of times your heart beats per minute. Your resting heart rate may normally be between 60 and 90, depending on individual body differences. Exertion speeds up your heart rate, and so do coffee, some medications, and anxiety.

You can measure your heart rate by taking your pulse or by wearing a heart rate monitor. You can take your pulse at your wrist or neck. For feeling the pulse, your index and middle fingers are more sensitive than your thumb. Feel for your pulse by placing your fingertips at the base of the thumb of your opposite hand. If you can see the blue line of the radial artery, place your fingertips on it. Count the beats for exactly one minute.

Finding your neck pulse can be more difficult. Place an index and middle finger on either side of your windpipe and search until you find the pulse in your carotid artery. You have one on each side of your neck. When counting, don't press down too hard on the artery or you may slow the beat.

The most convenient and reliable heart rate monitor is the type that is attached by a thin chest strap and that transmits to a watchlike monitor worn on the wrist. You can tell your heart rate at a glance without stopping what you are doing, which is why I recommend it. A heart rate monitor can be purchased for about $60, with more elaborate models costing up to $400.

The traditional way to estimate your maximum heart rate is to subtract your age from 220. Thus, if you are 50 years old, your maximum heart rate is 170 ($220 - 50 = 170$). This is only an estimate, and a person's actual maximum heart rate may be as much as 15 beats faster or slower. In our example, your target range of exertion (50 to 85 percent of your maximum heart rate), is 85 to 145 heartbeats per minute:

$$170 \times 0.50 = 85 \qquad 170 \times 0.85 = 145$$

To find your actual exercising heart rate, you must pause while exercising and measure your heart rate—that is, take your pulse. If you find that your heart rate is still in the 80s, you know you are exerting yourself at a minimal level—just barely enough to count as heart-healthy exercise at all. On the other hand, if you have a pulse of 145, you are pushing yourself too hard and need to slow down in a hurry.

As your body becomes conditioned through exercise, you will notice that exertions take less effort. For example, an exertion that once raised your heartbeat to 120 may now raise it to only 110. Over time, the more you exercise, the more you can exert yourself without approaching your limit.

Whether you exercise or not, your physical condition is never static. Your body and health are always improving or getting worse. Much of the psychic reward of exercise is seeing your physical improvement.

Subtracting your age from 220 is only a rough formula to find your maximum heart rate. The Karvonen method is more accurate, if you are willing to do the math. Because it factors in your resting heart rate, the Karvonen method is regarded as more responsive to individual differences.

For example, if you are 50 years old and have a resting heart rate of 72 beats per minute, you would estimate your pulse target range as follows:

1. Subtract your age from 220: $220 - 50 = 170$
2. Subtract your resting heart rate from your estimated maximum heart rate: $170 - 72 = 98$
3. Multiply the result of step 2 by 50 percent and then add your resting heart rate: $(98 \times 0.50) + 72 = 121$
4. Multiply the result of step 2 by 85 percent and then add your resting heart rate: $(98 \times 0.85) + 72 = 155$

Your pulse target range according to the Karvonen method is 121 to 155. This contrasts with the earlier rough estimate of 85 to 145. The main difference for you is that the Karvonen method raises the minimum level of exertion needed to benefit your heart. But once more, you need to keep in mind that this is only an estimate. In real life, no matter how modest it is, any exercise benefits your body and heart.

Stress Reduction

At the Integrative Cardiology Center, I always recommend combining moderate exercise with relaxation techniques or other methods of reducing stress. Yoga is an increasingly proven way to relax. It also has a multitude of other health benefits. You will not be expected to assume advanced postures when you start. Even so, there are health benefits at this stage. Experienced instructors can help you with alternative postures as you work your way toward more advanced routines. Gardening or woodworking works just as well. These are physical activities that you become so involved in, you don't notice time passing. This is what makes them, in a sense, meditative activities. This meditative quality takes you out of yourself, relaxes you, and reduces stress.

At the clinic, I put many stress-reducing techniques to use. Although this book is not the place to describe them, I want to say how important I think they are. Don't rely on diet and exercise alone. Looking after your emotional and spiritual welfare can be equally important to your heart health.

Afterword:
The Test You Think You Took
But Were Not Given

O f all the possible blood tests to check cardiovascular health, if only a couple could be taken, which would they be?

First, let me say that the more tests you take, the more reliable your results will be. One test result confirms or contradicts another. It might make sense to doubt one test result. But when three different tests all say the same thing, you need to listen. So, taking only a couple of tests is not a desirable thing to do. With that understood, which would they be?

I would choose the test that is an excellent predictor of cardiac events—CRP—and the test that best tells me how I stand and what action I need to take—LDL.

Your C-reactive protein level is without doubt an excellent predictor of heart attacks. As we know, it is a better predictor than

LDL cholesterol level, which was previously the best cardiac predictor we had. If your CPR is above 1, you need to take another test in three months. If the lower reading of the two CRP tests is above 3, you know that you have inflammation taking place in your body and that your heart health is threatened. Eat healthy. Reduce your waistline. Take moderate exercise, such as walking briskly, for at least thirty minutes each day. This should lower your CRP—and your LDL. If this does not work, your doctor may suggest a statin. Doctors don't know why statins lower CRPs along with LDLs, but they do.

Your low-density lipoprotein cholesterol level seems to deliver a simple message. We know that LDL ferries cholesterol to injury sites in artery walls. LDL is engulfed by macrophages and becomes oxidized in the artery walls, enlarging plaque. Your LDL level should be below 100.

But is that value too high? If there is a change, you can be sure the number will be revised downward, not upward. New recommendations may be for a ceiling of 70, instead of 100.

With the importance of LDL levels, it may come as a surprise to many that their LDL was not *directly* measured, but simply calculated. This is how it is done. Your total cholesterol level is the sum of your HDL, LDL, and VLDL. Your VLDL is calculated as one-fifth of your triglyceride level. This is why it is so important to fast for eight to twelve hours before giving a blood sample, because your triglyceride level is much more responsive to food intake than any other lipid level.

With direct tests of only your total cholesterol, HDL, and triglycerides, your LDL is calculated as follows (when your triglyceride level is below 250):

$$LDL = total\ cholesterol - HDL - (triglycerides/5)$$

A direct test of LDL costs about $150. If an accurate result can be calculated from other direct tests, it makes economic sense to use the calculated result. A direct test, which includes a measurement of particle size, may be covered by your medical insurance company if your calculated LDL level is high. How accurate is the calculated LDL result? A direct LDL test result rarely coincides with a calculated one. When a patient has both, the direct test result is usually higher than the calculated result. The spread between them can be as much as 20.

For someone with an LDL at or close to the desirable ceiling value, a calculated result can be dangerously misleading. Bill, who has had a mild heart attack, feels he can cheat on his diet a little and maybe enjoy an occasional cigarette, since his LDL is at 99. If Bill had a direct LDL test, he might learn that in reality his LDL is 115 and the particle size is small, which means an even higher risk. In that case, Bill needs more dieting and exercise, not less.

How can you tell whether your LDL level was a direct measurement or simply calculated? Divide your triglyceride level by 5, add that sum to your HDL, and subtract both from your total cholesterol level. If the arithmetic works out neatly, chances are you are reading calculator results.

Your calculated LDL level may be well below the desirable ceiling value of 100—it should be! But in reality you may not have as much of a safety zone as you think. Your direct LDL may be higher by 10. And perhaps the desirable ceiling value should be lower by 30.

Does it matter? Very much, in my opinion. You may remember the many times I have recommended trimming your waistline through healthy eating and moderate exercise. That's only another way of saying, lower your LDL.

Your heart and blood circulation are a complex system. Inflammatory markers, lipids, lipoproteins, blood-clotting proteins, homocysteine, and insulin, among other agents, have beneficial roles to play when their levels are optimal—and harmful roles when their levels become elevated. They operate independently as risk factors or they cooperate with one another and raise the risk level synergistically.

We need more than one dial on the dashboard. The seven new tests for heart health described in this book can be seen as seven more dials, giving you seven new sources of information. Any one of these sources can give you advance warning, providing you with time to take preventive action against potential heart problems or to alleviate a problem that has already arrived.

Resources

Information on Many Aspects of Cardiovascular Health

American Heart Association
7272 Greenville Avenue
Dallas, TX 75231
(800) 242-8721
www.americanheart.org
The American Heart Association issued new guidelines to help women prevent heart attacks and strokes. Phone 1-888-MYHEART (1-888-694-3278).

Centers for Disease Control and Prevention
Division of Nutrition and Physical Activity and Health Promotion
7440 Buford Highway, NE-MS/K-24
Atlanta, GA 30341-3717
770-488-5820
www.cdc.gov/nccdphp/dnpa

You can have the CDC calculate your body mass index (BMI) online by going to www.cdc.gov/nccdphp/dnpa/bmi.

National Cholesterol Education Program
National Heart, Lung and Blood Institute Health Information Center
P.O. Box 30105
Bethesda, MD 20824-0105
www.nhlbi.nih.gov/guidelines/cholesterol/atp_iii.htm

Information on Nutrition

American Dietetic Association: www.eatright.org. Click on "Food & Nutrition Information."

Center for Science in the Public Interest: www.cspinet.org.

Healthatoz.com. Click on "Lifestyles" and then on "Nutrition."

U.S. Department of Agriculture: www.usda.gov/fnutrition.html

Information on Women's Health Issues

American Heart Association: www.women.americanheart.org

American Medical Women's Association: www.amwa-doc.org

General information: www.ivillage.com

Microsoft Network: www.womencentral.msn.com

National Coalition for Women with Heart Disease: www.womenheart.org

National Women's Health Resource Center: www.healthywomen.org

General Information

www.ahcpr.gov
www.healthology.com
www.health.netscape.com
www.health.yahoo.com
www.heartpoint.com
www.mayoclinic.com

www.netwellness.org
www.nhlbi.nih.gov
www.noah-health.org
www.rxlist.com
www.webmd.com

References and Background Reading

1. A New Look at Heart Disease

Jack Challem, *The Inflammation Syndrome,* New York: Wiley, 2003.

Daniel G. Hackam and Sonia S. Anand, "Emerging Risk Factors for Atherosclerotic Vascular Disease," *JAMA,* 290:932–940, 2003.

Peter Libby et al., "Inflammation and Atherosclerosis," *Circulation,* 105:1135–1143, 2002.

Thomas A. Pearson et al., "Markers of Inflammation and Cardiovascular Disease," *Circulation,* 197:499–511, 2003.

Russell Ross, "Atherosclerosis—An Inflammatory Disease," *N. Engl. J. Med.,* 340(2):115–126, 1999.

2. Coronary Artery Disease Risk Factors

Burton Berkson and Jack Challem, *Syndrome X: The Complete Nutritional Program to Prevent and Reverse Insulin Resistance,* New York: Wiley, 2001.

Gerald M. Reaven, *Insulin Resistance: The Metabolic Syndrome X*, Totowa, NJ: Humana, 1999.

Gerald M. Reaven, *Syndrome X, the Silent Killer: The New Heart Disease Risk*, New York: Fireside, 2001.

Stuart D. Rosen et al., "Silent Ischemia as a Central Problem: Regional Brain Activation Compared in Silent and Painful Myocardial Ischemia," *Ann. Int. Med.*, 124:939–949, 1996.

Neil Schneiderman et al., "Health Psychology: Psychosocial and Biobehavioral Aspects of Chronic Disease Management," *Annu. Rev. Psychol.*, 52:555–580, 2001.

3. Women's Heart Risks

K. W. Clarke et al., "Do Women with Acute Myocardial Infarction Receive the Same Treatment as Men?" *BMJ*, 309:563–566, 1994.

Pamela S. Douglas and Geoffrey S. Ginsburg, "The Evaluation of Chest Pain in Women," *N. Engl. J. Med.*, 334(20):1311–1315, 1996.

Harvard Women's Health Watch, monthly.

Robin Marantz Henig, "Taking Care of Everybody But Herself," *The New York Times*, June 24, 2001.

C. W. Hogue Jr. et al., "Sex Differences in Neurological Outcomes and Mortality After Cardiac Surgery," *Circulation*, 103(17):2133–2137, 2001.

Lori Mosca et al., "Cardiovascular Disease in Women," *Circulation*, 96:2468–2482, 1997.

Morris Notelovitz and Diana Tonnessen, *The Essential Heart Book for Women*, New York: St. Martin's Press, 1996.

The PDR Family Guide to Women's Health and Prescription Drugs, Montvale, NJ: Medical Economics, 1994.

L. Pilote and M. A. Hlatky, "Attitudes of Women Toward Hormone Therapy and Prevention of Heart Disease," *Amer. Heart J.*, 129:1237–1238, 1995.

A. K. Sullivan et al., "Chest Pain in Women: Clinical, Investigative, and Prognostic Features," *BMJ*, 308:883–886, 1994.

Nanette Kass Wenger, "Coronary Heart Disease: An Older Woman's Major Health Risk," *BMJ*, 315:1085–1090, 1997.

Nanette Kass Wenger, "The High Risk of CHD for Women: Understanding Why Prevention Is Crucial," *Medscape Women's Health*, 1(11):6, 1996.

Ron Winslow, "New Guidelines Tackle Women's Health Risks," *The Wall Street Journal*, Feb. 5, 2004.

4. Why Knowing Your Cholesterol Level Isn't Enough

"The End of Heart Disease" (special issue), *U.S. News & World Report*, Dec. 1, 2003.

The Harvard Medical School Family Health Guide, New York: Simon & Schuster, 2000.

Stephen Holt, *The Natural Way to a Healthy Heart: Lessons from Alternative and Conventional Medicine*, New York: Evans, 1999.

Johns Hopkins Complete Guide for Preventing and Reversing Heart Disease, New York: Prima/Random House, 1998.

Thomas A. Pearson et al., "Markers of Inflammation and Cardiovascular Disease," *Circulation*, 197:499–511, 2003.

James M. Rippe, *The Healthy Heart for Dummies*, Foster City, CA: IDG Books, 2000.

5. C-reactive Protein Test

Christine M. Albert et al., "Prospective Study of C-reactive Protein, Homocysteine, and Plasma Lipid Levels as Predictors of Sudden Cardiac Death," *Circulation*, 105:2595–2599, 2002.

Mary S. Beattie et al., "C-reactive Protein and Ischemia in Users and Nonusers of Beta-Blockers and Statins," *Circulation*, 107:245–250, 2003.

Jane E. Brody, "Hunt for Heart Disease Tracks a New Suspect," *The New York Times*, Jan. 6, 2004.

D. Chew et al., "Effect of Clopidogrel Added to Aspirin Before Percutaneous Coronary Intervention on the Risk Associated with C-reactive Protein," *Am. J. Cardiol.*, 88:672–674, 2001.

F. M. Grace and B. Davies, "Raised Concentrations of C-reactive Protein in Anabolic Steroid Using Bodybuilders," *Br. J. Sports Med.*, 38(1):97–98, 2004.

Daniel G. Hackam and Sonia S. Anand, "Emerging Risk Factors for Atherosclerotic Vascular Disease: A Critical Review of the Evidence," *JAMA*, 290:932–940, 2003.

S. M. Haffner et al., "Effect of Rosiglitazone Treatment on Nontraditional

Markers of Cardiovascular Disease in Patients with Type 2 Diabetes Mellitus," *Circulation,* 106:679–684, 2002.

Dean J. Kereiakes, "The Fire That Burns Within: C-reactive Protein," *Circulation,* 107:373–374, 2003.

Peter Libby et al., "Inflammation and Atherosclerosis," *Circulation,* 105:1135–1143, 2002.

A. M. Linkoff et al., "Abciximab Suppresses the Rise in Levels of Circulating Inflammatory Markers After Percutaneous Coronary Revascularization," *Circulation,* 104:163–167, 2001.

H. K. Meier-Ewert et al., "Effect of Sleep Loss on C-reactive Protein, an Inflammatory Marker of Cardiovascular Risk," *J. Am. Coll. Cardiol.,* 43(4):678–683, 2004.

Michele Meyer, "Red Hot Revelations," *AARP Bulletin,* October 2003.

S. E. Nissen et al., "Statin Therapy, LDL Cholesterol, C-reactive Protein, and Coronary Artery Disease," *N. Engl. J. Med.,* 352(1):29–38, 2005.

Tara Parker-Pope, "A Number That Can Change Your Life: Simple Heart Test Leads to Better Habits," *The Wall Street Journal,* Aug. 5, 2003.

Thomas A. Pearson et al., "Markers of Inflammation and Cardiovascular Disease," *Circulation,* 107:499–511, 2003.

Paul M. Ridker, "Should Statin Therapy Be Considered for Patients with Elevated C-reactive Protein?" *Eur. Heart J.,* 22:2135–2137, 2001.

Paul M. Ridker et al., "C-reactive Protein Levels and Outcomes After Statin Therapy," *N. Engl. J. Med.,* 352(1):20–28, 2005.

Paul M. Ridker et al., "Clinical Application of C-reactive Protein for Cardiovascular Disease Detection and Prevention," *Circulation,* 107:363–369, 2003.

Paul M. Ridker et al., "Comparison of C-reactive Protein and Low-density Lipoprotein Cholesterol Levels in the Prediction of First Cardiovascular Events," *N. Engl. J. Med.,* 347(20):1557–1565, 2002.

W. L. Roberts et al., "Evaluation of Nine Automated High Sensitivity C-reactive Protein Methods," *Clin. Chem.,* 47:418–423, 2001.

Ron Winslow, "New Heart Test Gets Major Backing," *The Wall Street Journal,* Jan. 28, 2003.

Ron Winslow, "Study Confirms Better Predictor of Heart Risk," *The Wall Street Journal,* Nov. 14, 2002.

Edward T. H. Yeh and James T. Willerson, "Coming of Age of C-reactive Protein," *Circulation*, 107:370–372, 2003.

6. Fibrinogen Test

M. Acevedo et al., "Elevated Fibrinogen and Homocysteine Levels Enhance the Risk of Mortality in Patients from a High-Risk Preventive Cardiology Clinic," *Arterioscler. Thromb. Vasc. Biol.*, 22:1042–1045, 2002.

L. Doweik et al., "Fibrinogen Predicts Mortality in High-Risk Patients with Peripheral Artery Disease," *Eur. J. Vasc. Endovasc. Surg.*, 26(4): 381–386, 2003.

Daniel G. Hackam and Sonia S. Anand, "Emerging Risk Factors for Atherosclerotic Vascular Disease: A Critical Review of the Evidence," *JAMA*, 290:932–940, 2003.

B. R. Jaeger and C. A. Labarrere, "Fibrinogen and Atherothrombosis: Vulnerable Plaque or Vulnerable Patient?" *Herz*, 28(6):530–538, 2003.

B. Kerlin et al., "Cause-Effect Relation Between Hyperfibrinogenemia and Vascular Disease," *Blood*, 103(5):1728–1734, 2004.

M. Kozlowska-Wojciechowska et al., "Impact of Margarine Enriched with Plant Sterols on Blood Lipids, Platelet Function, and Fibrinogen Level in Young Men," *Metabolism*, 52(11):1373–1378, 2003.

T. Meade et al., "Bezafibrate in Men with Lower Extremity Arterial Disease: Randomised Controlled Trial," *BMJ*, 325:1139, 2002.

Thomas A. Pearson et al., "Markers of Inflammation and Cardiovascular Disease," *Circulation*, 107:499–511, 2003.

V. Schechner et al., "Significant Dominance of Fibrinogen Over Immunoglobulins, C-reactive Protein, Cholesterol and Triglycerides in Maintaining Increased Red Blood Cell Adhesiveness/Aggregation in the Peripheral Venous Blood: A Model in Hypercholesterolaemic Patients," *Eur. J. Clin. Invest.*, 33(11):955–961, 2003.

J. S. Sidhu et al., "The Effect of Rosiglitazone, a Peroxisome Proliferator-Activated Receptor-Gamma Agonist, on Markers of Endothelial Cell Activation, C-reactive Protein, and Fibrinogen Levels in Nondiabetic Coronary Artery Disease Patients," *J. Am. Coll. Cardiol.*, 42(10):1757–1763, 2003.

S. G. Wannamethee et al., "Physical Activity and Hemostatic and Inflammatory Variables in Elderly Men," *Circulation*, 105:1785, 2002.

M. Woodward et al., "Does Sticky Blood Predict a Sticky End? Associations of Blood Viscosity, Haematocrit and Fibrinogen with Mortality in the West of Scotland," *Br. J. Haematol.*, 122(4):645–650, 2003.

7. Homocysteine Test

Jane E. Brody, "Health Sleuths Assess Homocysteine as Culprit," *The New York Times*, June 13, 2000.

X. Gao et al., "Plasma C-reactive Protein and Homocysteine Concentrations Are Related to Frequent Fruit and Vegetable Intake in Hispanic and Non-Hispanic White Elders," *J. Nutr.*, 134(4):913–918, 2004.

R. F. Gillum, "Distribution of Total Serum Homocysteine and Its Association with Parental History and Cardiovascular Risk Factors at Ages 12–16 Years: The Third National Health and Nutrition Examination Survey," *Ann. Epidemiol.*, 14(3):229–233, 2004.

Daniel G. Hackam and Sonia S. Anand, "Emerging Risk Factors for Atherosclerotic Vascular Disease: A Critical Review of the Evidence," *JAMA*, 290:932–940, 2003.

Kilmer S. McCully, *The Homocysteine Revolution*, New Canaan, CT: Keats, 1997.

Amy Dockser Marcus, "Folic Acid's Benefits Go Beyond Birth," *The Wall Street Journal*, March 2, 2004.

S. S. Moselhy and S. H. Demerdash, "Plasma Homocysteine and Oxidative Stress in Cardiovascular Disease, *Dis. Markers.*, 19(1):27–31, 2003.

Russell Ross, "Atherosclerosis: An Inflammatory Disease," *N. Engl. J. Med.*, 340(2):115–126, 1999.

David A. Snowdon et al., "Serum Folate and the Severity of Atrophy of the Neocortex in Alzheimer Disease: Findings from the Nun Study," *Am. J. Clin. Nutr.*, 71:993–998, 2000.

J. D. Spence, "Patients with Atherosclerotic Vascular Disease: How Low Should Plasma Homocysteine Go?" *Am. J. Cardiovasc. Drugs*, 1(2): 85–89, 2001.

James F. Toole et al., "Lowering Homocysteine in Patients with Ischemic Stroke to Prevent Recurrent Stroke, Myocardial Infraction, and Death," *JAMA*, 291:565–575, 2004.

K. R. Vincent et al., "Homocysteine and Lipoprotein Levels Following Resistance Training in Older Adults," *Prev. Cardiol.*, 6(4):197–203, 2003.

D. E. Zylberstein et al., "Serum Homocysteine in Relation to Mortality and Morbidity from Coronary Heart Disease: A 24-Year Follow-up of the Population Study of Women in Gothenburg," *Circulation*, 109(5):601–606, 2004.

8. Fasting Insulin Test

John P. Cooke, "Endothelium-Derived Factors and Peripheral Vascular Disease," *Cardiovasc. Clin.*, 22:3–17, 1992.

H. O. Steinberg et al., "Obesity/Insulin Resistance Is Associated with Endothelial Dysfunction: Implications for the Syndrome of Insulin Resistance," *J. Clin. Invest.*, 97:2601–2610, 1996.

Samuel S. Thatcher, *PCOS—Polycystic Ovary Syndrome: The Hidden Epidemic*, Indianapolis: Perspectives Press, 2000.

J. G. Yu et al., "The Effect of Thiazolidinediones on Plasma Adiponectin Levels in Normal, Obese, and Diabetic Subjects," *Diabetes*, 51:2968–2974, 2002.

9. Ferritin Test

Michael Haap et al., "Association of High Serum Ferritin Concentration with Glucose Intolerance and Insulin Resistance in Healthy People," *Ann. Int. Med.*, 139(10):869–871, 2003.

Rui Jiang et al., "Body Iron Stores in Relation to Risk of Type 2 Diabetes in Apparently Healthy Women," *JAMA*, 291(6):711–717, 2004.

A. G. Mainous III et al., "Association of Ferritin and Lipids with C-Reactive Protein," *Am. J. Cardiol.*, 93(5):559–562, 2004.

Laura E. Murray-Kolb et al., "Women with Low Iron Stores Absorb Iron from Soybeans," *Am. J. Clin. Nutr.*, 77(1):180–184, 2003.

Jukka Salonen et al., "High Stored Iron Levels Are Associated with Excess Risk of Myocardial Infarction in Eastern Finnish Men," *Circulation*, 86:803–811, 1992.

T. P. Tuomainen et al., "Serum Ferritin Concentration Is Associated with Plasma Levels of Cholestrol Oxidation Products in Man," *Free Radic. Biol. Med.*, 35(8):922–928, 2003.

M. J. Williams, "Ferritin and Cardiovascular Risk," *Atherosclerosis,* 167(1):171, 2003.

S. A. You et al., "Proteomic Approach to Coronary Atherosclerosis Shows Ferritin Light Chain as a Significant Marker: Evidence Consistent with Iron Hypothesis in Atherosclerosis," *Physiol. Genomics,* 13(1): 25–30, 2003.

10. Lipoprotein(a) Test

Abraham A. Ariyo et al., "Lp(a) Lipoprotein, Vascular Disease, and Mortality in the Elderly," *N. Engl. J. Med.,* 349(22):2103–2115, 2003.

E. Campos, "Lipoprotein(a): Its Importance as an Additional Atherosclerosis Marker," *Acta Med. Port.,* 10(1):87–93, 2003.

A. Dirisamer and K. Widhalm, "Lipoprotein(a) as a Potent Risk Indicator for Early Cardiovascular Disease," *Acta Paediatr.,* 92(10):1226–1227, 2002.

A. Gonzalez-Requejo et al., "Lipoprotein(a) and Cardiovascular Risk Factors in a Cohort of 6-Year-Old Children: The Rivas-Vaciamadrid Study," *Eur. J. Pediatr.,* 162(9):572–575, 2003.

Daniel G. Hackam and Sonia S. Anand, "Emerging Risk Factors for Atherosclerotic Vascular Disease: A Critical Review of the Evidence," *JAMA,* 290:932–940, 2003.

E. D. Harris, "Lipoprotein(a): A Predictor of Atherosclerotic Disease," *Nutr. Rev.,* 55(3):61–64, 1997.

F. Hartgens et al., "Effects of Androgenic-Anabolic Steroids on Apolipoproteins and Lipoprotein(a)," *Br. J. Sports Med.,* 38(3): 253–259, 2004.

T. Iwamoto et al., "Long-Term Effects of Lipoprotein(a) on Carotid Atherosclerosis in Elderly Japanese," *J. Gerontol. A. Biol. Sci. Med. Sci.,* 59(1):62–67, 2004.

B. Jelakovic et al., "Lipoprotein(a): A Mysterious Factor in Atherogenesis," *Lijec. Vjesn.* (Croatia), 124(11–12):366–371, 2002.

A. Kalia, "Correlation of Lipoprotein(a) and Ischemic Heart Disease," *Orv. Hetil.* (Hungary), 143(47):2625–2629, 2002.

M. Kubo et al., "Contribution of Lp(a) to the Occurrence of Vascular Diseases: Correlation of Several Risk Factors Including Diabetes Mellitus," *J. Atheroscler. Thromb.,* 2(Suppl. 1):S22–S25, 1995.

A. Laraqui et al., "Homocysteine, Lipoprotein(a): Risk Factors for Coronary Heart Disease," *Ann. Biol. Clin.* (Paris), 60(5):549–557, 2002.

G. Lippi and G. Guidi, "Lipoprotein(a): An Emerging Cardiovascular Risk Factor," *Crit. Rev. Clin. Lab. Sci.*, 40(1):1–42, 2003.

S. M. Marcovina et al., "Report of the National Heart, Lung, and Blood Institute Workshop on Lipoprotein(a) and Cardiovascular Disease: Recent Advances and Future Directions," *Clin. Chem.*, 49(11):1785–1796, 2003.

S. M. Marcovina and M. L. Koschinsky, "Evaluation of Lipoprotein(a) as a Prothrombotic Factor: Progress from Bench to Bedside," *Curr. Opin. Lipidol.*, 14(4):361–366, 2003.

M. Miyao et al., "Lipoprotein(a) as a Risk Factor for Cardiovascular Disease in Elderly Patients with Diabetes," *Nippon Ronen Igakkai Zasshi*, 34(3):185–191, 1997.

M. B. Nielsen et al., "In Vivo Transfer of Lipoprotein(a) into Human Atherosclerotic Carotid Arterial Intima," *Arterioscler. Thromb. Vasc. Biol.*, 17(5):905–911, 1997.

A. de la Pena-Diaz et al., "Functional Approach to Investigate Lp(a) in Ischaemic Heart and Cerebral Disease," *Eur. J. Clin. Invest.*, 33(2): 99–105, 2003.

Mathias Rath and Linus Pauling, "Immunological Evidence for the Accumulation of Lipoprotein(a) in the Atherosclerotic Lesion of the Hypoascorbemic Guinea Pig," *Proc. Natl. Acad. Sci. USA*, 87:9388–9390, 1990.

N. Rifai et al., "Apolipoprotein(a) Size and Lipoprotein(a) Concentration and Future Risk of Angina Pectoris with Evidence of Severe Coronary Atherosclerosis in Men: The Physicians' Health Study," *Clin. Chem.*, May 20, 2004.

J. H. Stein and R. S. Rosenson, "Lipoprotein Lp(a) Excess and Coronary Heart Disease," *Arch. Intern. Med.*, 157(11):1170–1176, 1997.

H. D. Wu et al., "High Lipoprotein(a) Levels and Small Apolipoprotein(a) Sizes Are Associated with Endothelial Dysfunction in a Multiethnic Cohort," *J. Am. Coll. Cardiol.*, 43(10):1828–1833, 2004.

11. Calcium Heart Scan

Thomas M. Burton, "New Evidence Bolsters Use of Heart Scans," *The Wall Street Journal,* Jan. 14, 2004.

Philip Greenland et al., "Coronary Artery Calcium Score Combined with Framingham Score for Risk Prediction in Asymptomatic Individuals," *JAMA*, 291:210–215, 2004.

Larry Katzenstein, "It's Good in Your Bones, Bad in Your Arteries," *The New York Times*, Sept. 22, 2003.

George T. Kondos et al., "Electron-Beam Tomography Coronary Artery Calcium and Cardiac Events," *Circulation*, 107:2571–2576, 2003.

12. A New Look at the Old Tests

"A Statin Backlash," *The Wall Street Journal*, Jan. 26, 2004.

ALLHAT Collaborative Research Group, "Major Outcomes in High-Risk Hypertensive Patients Randomized to Angiotensin-Converting Enzyme Inhibitor or Calcium Channel Blocker Vs. Diuretic," *JAMA*, 288:2981–2997, 2002.

Zachary T. Bloomgarden, "Diabetes and Hypertension," *Diabetes Care*, 24(9):1679–1684, 2001.

Zachary T. Bloomgarden, "Inflammation and Insulin Resistance," *Diabetes Care*, 26(5):1619–1623, 2003.

"Britain to Approve Cholesterol Drugs for OTC Sale," *The Wall Street Journal*, May 11, 2004.

Aram V. Chobanian et al., "The Seventh Report of the Joint National Committee on Prevention, Detection, Evaluation, and Treatment of High Blood Pressure," *JAMA*, 289:2560–2572, 2003.

Michael R. Ehrenstein et al., "Statins for Atherosclerosis—As Good As It Gets?" *N. Engl. J. Med.*, 352(1):73–75, 2005.

Denise Grady, "U.S. Guidelines Reassess Blood Pressure," *The New York Times*, May 15, 2003.

Scott M. Grundy et al., "Implications of Recent Clinical Trials for the National Cholesterol Education Program Adult Treatment Panel III Guidelines," *Circulation*, 110:227–239, 2004.

Beth Howard, "Fat Chance," *Remedy*, Winter 2003, pp. 30–36.

Nancy Ann Jeffrey, "Home Cholesterol Check," *The Wall Street Journal*, Feb. 27, 2004.

Gina Kolata, "Cholesterol Study Offers Hope for a Bold Therapy," *The New York Times*, Nov. 5, 2003.

Gina Kolata, "Just How Low Can You Go? A Cholesterol Challenge," *The New York Times,* Dec. 2, 2003.

Gina Kolata, "Scientists Begin to Question Benefit of 'Good' Cholesterol," *The New York Times,* March 15, 2004.

Gina Kolata, "Study of Two Cholesterol Drugs Finds One Halts Heart Disease," *The New York Times,* Nov. 13, 2003.

Michael D. Lemonick, "Drano for the Heart," *Time,* Nov. 17, 2003.

Peter Libby et al., "Inflammation and Atherosclerosis," *Circulation,* 105:1135–1143, 2002.

Eric Nagourney, "A Season for High Cholesterol," *The New York Times,* May 4, 2004.

National Cholesterol Education Program, *Third Report of the Expert Panel on Detection, Evaluation, and Treatment of High Blood Cholesterol in Adults (Adult Treatment Panel III): Executive Summary,* www.nhlbi.nih.gov/guidelines/cholesterol/atp_iii.htm.

Steven E. Nissen et al., "Effect of Recombinant ApoA-I Milano on Coronary Atherosclerosis in Patients with Acute Coronary Syndromes," *JAMA,* 290:2292–2300, 2003.

David Noonan, "You Want Statins with That?," *Newsweek,* July 14, 2003.

Tara Parker-Pope, "Cholesterol Drugs May Cause Side Effects That Mimic Aging," *The Wall Street Journal,* Dec. 16, 2002.

Lisa Sanders, "Shortness of Breath, High Cholesterol, No Fever or Cough," *The New York Times Magazine,* Dec. 7, 2003.

Jan A. Staessen et al., "Antihypertensive Treatment Based on Blood Pressure Measurement at Home or in the Physician's Office," *JAMA,* 291:955–964, 2004.

Ron Winslow, "New HDL Drug Shows Promise in Heart Study," *The Wall Street Journal,* Nov. 5, 2003.

Ron Winslow, "Study Signals How Low to Go on Cholesterol," *The Wall Street Journal,* Nov. 13, 2003.

Ron Winslow, "The New Rules of Blood Pressure," *The Wall Street Journal,* May 15, 2003.

13. Supporting Heart Health with Lifestyle

Anjana Ahuja, "A Fitter, Healthier World? Fat Chance," *The Times* (London), May 21, 2003.

Shelly Branch, "Is Food the Next Tobacco?" *The Wall Street Journal*, June 13, 2002.

C. Leigh Broadhurst, *Diabetes: Prevention and Cure*, New York: Kensington, 1999.

Jane E. Brody, "Cholesterol: When It's Good, It's Very, Very Good," *The New York Times*, July 15, 2003.

Jane E. Brody, "The Widening of America, or How Size 4 Became Size 0," *The New York Times*, Jan. 20, 2004.

Mark Francis Cohen, "What's Worse Than Sugar?," *AARP Bulletin*, April 2004.

Greg Critser, *Fat Land: How Americans Became the Fattest People in the World*, Boston: Houghton Mifflin, 2003.

"Death Rate from Obesity Gains Fast on Smoking," *The New York Times*, March 10, 2004.

David Derbyshire, "Obesity Will Top Smoking as Main Cause of Cancer," *Daily Telegraph* (London), April 6, 2004.

Denise Grady, "Liposuction Doesn't Offer Health Benefit, Study Finds," *The New York Times*, June 17, 2004.

Denise Grady, "More Support for Eating Fatty Fish," *The New York Times*, April 10, 2002.

Sarah Lueck, "Winning by Losing," *The Wall Street Journal*, Oct. 21, 2003.

Betsy McKay, "Politicians Tackle Weighty Issues," *The Wall Street Journal*, Nov. 16, 2003.

Betsy McKay, "Who You Calling Fat?" *The Wall Street Journal*, July 23, 2002.

Tara Parker-Pope, "The Diet That Works," *The Wall Street Journal*, April 22, 2003.

Richard Perez-Pena, "Obesity on Rise in New York Public Schools," *The New York Times*, July 9, 2003.

Physical Activity and Health: A Report of the Surgeon General, www.cdc.gov/nccdphp/sgr/chapcon.htm.

Suzanne Schlosberg and Liz Neporent, *Fitness for Dummies*, Foster City, CA: IDG Books, 2000.

Elaine Sciolino, "France, Seams Under Pressure, Remeasures Itself," *The New York Times*, April 25, 2003.

Kelly K. Spors, "Don't Just Sit There," *The Wall Street Journal*, Oct. 21, 2003.

Peg Tyre, "In a Race Against Time," *Newsweek*, Jan. 19, 2004.

Glossary

Adult-onset diabetes: See *Type 2 diabetes*.

Angina pectoris: A pain in the center of the chest that worsens with activity and eases with rest. It is caused by plaque impeding blood flow through one or more coronary arteries, resulting in an insufficient blood supply to part of the heart muscle.

Antioxidant: A substance capable of combining with an oxygen free radical and making a harmless end product. The antioxidant thus prevents the free radical from potentially making a substance harmful to the body by combining with another substance.

Arteriosclerosis: Thickening of the arterial wall with age or high blood pressure. The term can also refer to calcification of the arterial wall with age. Often used in the same sense as "atherosclerosis."

Artery: A blood vessel carrying oxygenated blood from the heart to the body.

Atherosclerosis: Development of plaque in the inner wall of the arteries.

Bile acid sequestrant: A kind of cholesterol-lowering drug.

Body mass index (BMI): A ranking of recommended weight according to height. People with a BMI of 25 to 29 are regarded as overweight, and those with a BMI of 30 or more are obese. Those with a BMI below 18 are underweight.

C-reactive protein (CRP): An inflammatory marker and predictor of heart attacks, strokes, peripheral artery disease, and sudden cardiac death. This protein, manufactured by the liver, appears in the bloodstream once inflammation occurs and disappears shortly after inflammation subsides.

Calorie: For our purposes, a measurement of the energy-producing value in food when oxidized in the body. The higher a food's calorie count, the more activity required to use it up.

Carbohydrate: An organic compound composed of carbon, hydrogen, and oxygen. Fruits and vegetables are made up almost entirely of carbohydrates. All carbohydrates from food are converted by the body into blood glucose as a source of energy. Starches, simple sugars, and refined grains are the carbohydrates most rapidly converted by the body into blood glucose.

Cardiovascular: Having to do with the heart and blood circulation.

Cholesterol: A lipoprotein found in cell walls, nerve sheaths, all tissues, and blood. Manufactured by the liver, cholesterol is also absorbed from food—about 500 to 1,000 milligrams per day in the Western diet. It comes in the form of HDL, LDL, and VLDL.

Cholesterol level: This is understood to mean total cholesterol blood level, which is HDL+LDL+VLDL.

Cis fat: Fat with the natural bond structure. Processed foods may have their fats wholly or partly hydrogenated to change the cis to the trans bond structure, which has a longer shelf life. The trans structure is not a naturally occurring form, and our bodies are not adapted to digest it.

Coronary artery disease: Plaque formation in the walls of the coronary arteries, which supply blood to the heart muscle. The disease process is called "atherosclerosis." Plaque can restrict blood flow, resulting in angina pectoris. A blood clot on ruptured plaque can block a coronary artery, causing a heart attack. Also known as "coronary heart disease."

Endothelium: The single layer of sensitive cells that line the inside walls of arteries and veins, the heart, and lymphatic vessels.

Fat: An organic substance made up of fatty acids that can conveniently be thought of as body fat and dietary fat. Body fat (adipose tissue) is used to store energy and as a protective covering for internal organs. Units of body fat are called "triglycerides." Dietary fat comes in three kinds: saturated, polyunsaturated, and monounsaturated, so-called according to their ability to bond with other substances.

Fatty streak: A fatty streak is formed in the artery wall by foam cells and other blood cells that have engulfed foreign particles.

Ferritin: A protein that is the body's main way of storing the mineral iron. It is found in the blood and in all organs and tissues.

Fibrate: A kind of cholesterol-lowering drug.

Fibrinogen: A protein made by the liver that acts as an inflammatory marker in the blood. The fibrinogen level can increase fourfold in response to inflammation. Fibrinogen has a direct role in atherosclerosis by promoting and taking part in clot formation.

Foam cell: In artery wall plaque, a macrophage scavenger blood cell that becomes transformed when it engulfs an LDL particle.

Folic acid: B vitamin that is important in fetal development, nucleic acid formation, and other basic life processes. Also known as "folate."

Free radical: An atom or chemical group that can oxidize another substance by combining with it. The resulting product may or may not be harmful to the body.

Fructose: A simple sugar found in natural form in honey and some fruits. Table sugar (sucrose) is a mixture of fructose and glucose.

Glucose: A simple sugar that occurs naturally in grapes and a few other foods. The carbohydrates that we eat are converted to glucose in the blood, and our body cells consume it for energy.

Glucose intolerance: A state in which blood glucose regulation requires higher levels of insulin due to obesity and insulin resistance. It is often an intermediate step to type 2 diabetes.

Glycemic index: A ranking of carbohydrate foods according to their impact on blood glucose and insulin levels. Calories are not considered.

HDL: High-density lipoprotein ("good") cholesterol that transports cholesterol from the blood to the liver, where it is broken down.

Heart attack: Death of part of the heart muscle due to lack of blood supply from a blocked coronary artery. Also known as "acute myocardial infarction."

Homocysteine: A protein that acts as an inflammatory marker in the blood. Homocysteine also plays a direct role in atherosclerosis by damaging the cells lining the artery wall, stimulating the proliferation of smooth muscle cells in the artery wall, and acting as a source of free radicals for the oxidation of LDL. Homocysteine may also contribute to clot formation on ruptured plaque.

Hydrogenated food: Processed foods in which the natural cis bond structure of fats has been changed, through treatment with hydrogen, to the artificial trans structure, which has a longer shelf life.

Hypertension: High blood pressure.

Inflammation: The body's response to injury. The tissue affected may become red, swollen, hot, and painful. White blood cells attack foreign particles, such as bacteria. Acute inflammation is short-term because the cause of injury is brief and healing sets in. When the cause of injury remains present, chronic inflammation can result.

Inflammatory marker: A substance in the blood whose level is responsive to inflammation.

Insulin: A protein hormone secreted by cells of the pancreas. It controls blood glucose, sending some to the cell to be consumed for energy and storing some for future use in the liver and adipose tissue.

Insulin resistance: Increasing lack of sensitivity on the part of cells to insulin's regulation of blood glucose. With insulin resistance, it takes a higher insulin level to keep blood glucose at a normal level. The higher insulin level damages the body. Insulin resistance is the cause of type 2 diabetes and a major cause of the metabolic syndrome.

Ischemia: A lack of blood due to blockage or constriction of an artery.

LDL: Low-density lipoprotein ("bad") cholesterol transports cholesterol through the blood to cells. It plays an important part in atherosclerosis.

Leukocyte: See *White blood cell.*

Lipid: One of a group of fatty compounds, insoluble in water, that can store energy, vitamins, and fatty acids. Fats and steroids are lipids.

Lipoprotein: A particle formed from the combination of a lipid and a protein. Cholesterol is a well-known example.

Macrophage: A large scavenger blood cell that engulfs foreign particles. It is closely related to the monocyte. Macrophages engulf LDL particles inside plaque in the artery wall.

Metabolic syndrome: The simultaneous occurrence of multiple cardiac risk factors that operate synergistically to raise the risk level. Insulin resistance and obesity are the basic risk factors that cause the syndrome. The syndrome can also include high total cholesterol, high LDL, low HDL, high triglycerides, high blood pressure, glucose intolerance, and type 2 diabetes. Also known as "syndrome X."

Monocyte: A white blood cell that ingests foreign particles in the bloodstream, such as bacteria and cell detritus.

Monounsaturated fat: A vegetable oil that is liquid at room temperature and often solidifies when refrigerated. Olive oil, peanut oil, and sesame oil are examples. They do not cause LDL and triglyceride blood levels to rise.

Myocardial infarction: See *Heart attack*.

Niacin: A powerful cholesterol-lowering agent, this B vitamin is available as a supplement without a prescription. Ingestion of excess amounts can cause liver damage. Also known as "nicotinic acid."

Obesity: The condition of people who weigh 20 percent or more above the weight recommended for their height. See also *Overweight*.

Omega fatty acid: A polyunsaturated fatty acid. Omega-3 fatty acids are found in cold-water marine fatty fish and in some seeds and nuts. Omega-6 fatty acids are found in many vegetable oils.

Overweight: The condition of people who weigh less than 20 percent above the weight recommended for their height. See also *Obesity*.

Plaque: In arteries, a deposit of cholesterol, other lipids, and cell detritus that builds in the inner wall. Plaque is often covered by a fibrous cap.

Polyunsaturated fat: Oils or fatty acids, the best known of which are the omega fatty acids. They do not cause LDL and triglyceride blood levels to rise.

Protein: A complex compound made up of amino acids. Proteins form the structures of muscles, tissues, and organs. They are also the major constituents of hormones and enzymes. The body uses amino acids, obtained from food or synthesized within itself, to manufacture proteins.

Risk factor: Something that increases your likelihood of being affected by a disorder.

Saturated fat: For our purposes, the fat found in animal meat, dairy products, and tropical vegetable oils. It raises LDL and triglyceride blood levels.

Statin: A kind of cholesterol-lowering drug.

Stroke: A response to blockage by a clot of an artery conveying blood to the brain. An ischemic stroke results when a clot forms and blocks the artery. An embolism is the result of artery blockage by a dislodged clot traveling in the blood.

Sucrose: Table sugar, a mixture of glucose and fructose.

Syndrome X: See *Metabolic syndrome*.

T cell: A kind of white blood cell important in cell-mediated immunity. Also known as a "T lymphocyte."

Total cholesterol level: See *Cholesterol level*.

Trans fat: In processed foods, fats with the natural cis bond structure treated with hydrogen to change it to the trans bond structure, which has a longer shelf life. The trans structure is not a naturally occurring form, and our bodies are not adapted to digest it.

Triglyceride: The form in which fat is stored in the body. It consists of glycerol combined with three fatty acid molecules.

Type 2 diabetes: A state in which blood glucose regulation requires higher levels of insulin, beyond glucose intolerance and due to obesity and insulin resistance. Also known as "adult-onset diabetes."

Vein: A blood vessel returning blood from the body to the heart and lungs so that it can be reoxygenated.

VLDL: Very low density lipoprotein cholesterol plays an important role in atherosclerosis. Its blood level is calculated as one-fifth of the triglyceride level.

White blood cell: A blood cell containing a nucleus, of which there are three main kinds, one being a monocyte. Also known as a "leukocyte."

Index

About the Author

Julius Torelli, M.D., is director of the Integrative Cardiology Center in High Point, North Carolina, between Greensboro and Winston-Salem. A board-certified cardiologist and internist, he served his internship and residency at the famed Cleveland Clinic in Ohio and was later awarded a Fellowship in Cardiovascular Disease there. He is a Fellow of the American College of Cardiology.

In his holistic practice at the Integrative Cardiology Center, Dr. Torelli provides heart patients with traditional and alternative therapies, assisted by licensed practitioners. He is married to Kimberly and has two children, Jessica and Daniel.

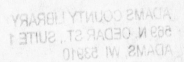